PENIS GENIUS

A QUIVER BOOK

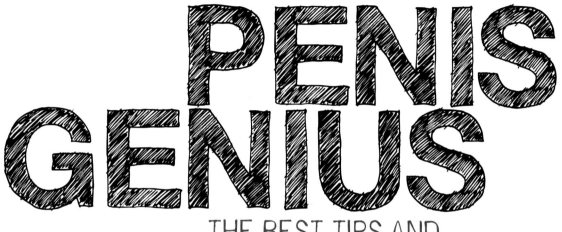

PENIS GENIUS

THE BEST TIPS AND TRICKS FOR WORKING HIS STICK

JORDAN LAROUSSE +
SAMANTHA SADE

Text © 2011 Yvonne Falvey Mihalik and Naomi Tepper
Illustrations © 2011 Quiver

First published in the USA in 2011 by
Quiver, a member of
Quayside Publishing Group
100 Cummings Center
Suite 406-L
Beverly, MA 01915-6101
www.quiverbooks.com

15 14 13 12 11   1 2 3 4 5

ISBN-13: 978-1-59233-460-5
ISBN-10: 1-59233-460-1

Library of Congress Cataloging-in-Publication Data available

Cover design by **Paul Burgess**
Book design by **Traffic**
Photography by **Holly Randall**

Printed and bound in **Singapore**

DEDICATION

To Tre', the ultimate lab partner
And always, to Joe

ODE TO THE PENIS

Life without penis would be a droopy, dreary place. There would be no dick jokes, erections, cock rings, or Caverject injections; there would be no place to hang your condom, no baby batter, and no big hard-ons. We wish to examine the cock's ins and outs, from its helmetlike head to the way it spouts. We say hooray for the penis in all of its glory, whether the size of a shrimp or eleven full stories.

CONTENTS

SOURCES FOR *PENIS GENIUS*

The information in this book comes from a variety of resources, including scientific journals, sex manuals (specifically, *Human Sexuality: Diversity in Contemporary America* by Bryan Strong and *Human Sexual Response* by William H. Masters and Virginia E. Johnson), personal interviews, plenty of hands-on trial and error, and two unscientific online surveys.

PENIS GENIUS SURVEYS

Using two anonymous online sex surveys, we gathered intimate information from approximately one thousand men and women. The first survey was open for several months in 2009 and the second for several months in 2010. Many participants found the survey links at OystersandChocolate.com, an online magazine for literary erotica, so we assume that most, if not all, respondents were at least sexually open enough to read erotic short stories. Many of the colorful quotes, statistics, graphs, and charts in this book are extrapolated from this survey, but please keep in mind that we are not scientists, nor are we professional statisticians.

Any identifying information attached to direct quotes, such as names, ages, and occupations, has been altered to protect the anonymity of the speaker.

References for the endnotes that appear throughout the text begin on page 163.

COMMON SENSE ON THE ROAD TO BECOMING A PENIS GENIUS

For many moons we researched the best bits of info for you in our effort to turn you into a bona fide penis genius. However, the advice given in this book is meant to be informative and entertaining; it is not meant to take the place of the professional advice of your physician or licensed sex therapist. Also, please be aware that you are fully responsible for anything you do or try in your sex life, so enjoy the tips in this book at your own risk. Be smart, be safe, be responsible—and *always* have fun.

WHY WE USE DIRTY WORDS

Plain and simple: We love them! There's just nothing like the properly placed dirty word, inside the bedroom or out. But moreover, we use words like *cock*, *pussy*, *balls*, and *fuck* because they properly and specifically describe what we're writing with the beauty of real-life terms. We don't say, "Please insert your penis into my vagina, honey," and we won't write that way, either.

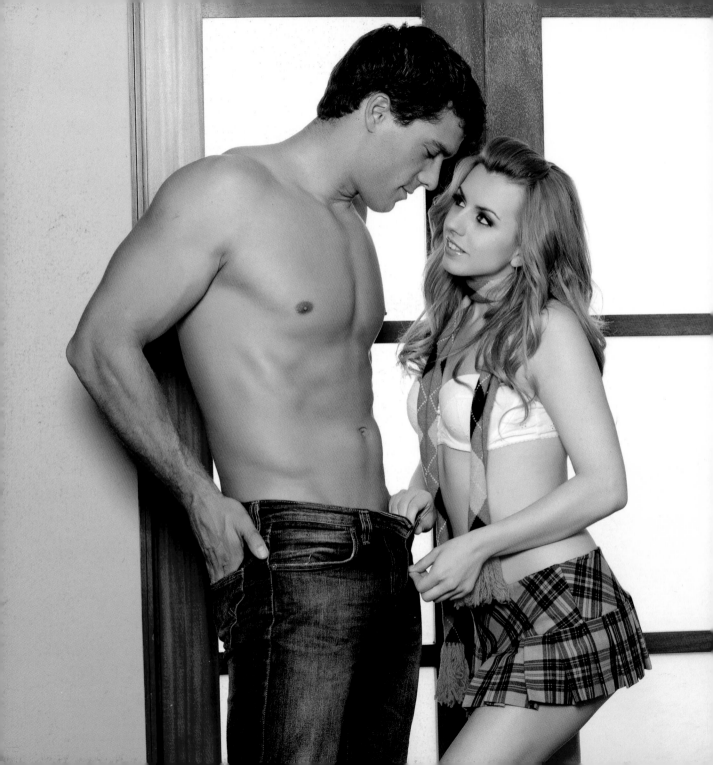

WHAT'S YOUR PENIS IQ?

Women like to think they know a thing or two about their man's package. However, those sexy little levers are a lot more complex than you might have ever imagined. It's our goal to turn you into a true penis genius. From anatomical facts to sexual tips, we guarantee this book will teach you fun and useful things about his dick that you never knew before.

Let's get started by taking a quiz designed to determine your penis IQ.

1. **What is the plural form of penis?**
   a. Penises (like vaginas)
   b. Peni (like cacti)
   c. Penes (like weenies)
   d. Both A and C
   e. All of the above

2. **Where is the frenulum?**
   a. At the base of the cock, where the shaft meets the testicles
   b. On the underside of the cock, where the shaft meets the head
   c. On the upper side of the cock, where the shaft meets the head
   d. Inside the scrotal sack; it's the tube that carries semen.

3. **What is the scrotal raphe?**
   a. A treasure trail that runs down the center of the scrotum; it's a good spot to lick.
   b. A tube inside the scrotum that transports semen
   c. The wrinkly skin of the scrotum
   d. The muscle that pulls the scrotum up to the body when cold

4. **What percentage of semen is made up of those little baby makers we call sperm?**
   a. 10 percent
   b. 69 percent
   c. 25 percent
   d. 1 percent

5. **If you are trying to get pregnant, what should your man avoid?**
   a. Hot tubs
   b. Strippers
   c. Alcohol
   d. Cigarettes
   e. All of the above

6. **Which of the following is true:**
   a. Semen is a good hair gel.
   b. Semen is good for your skin.
   c. Semen is a good source of vitamins.
   d. All of the above (save money on health and beauty products)
   e. None of the above (save it for the condom)

7. **When referring to sex positions, what is the Amazon?**
   a. When he comes on your back and lets the semen run down your spine like a river.
   b. A variation on doggy style: He bends you over the bed, you spread your legs wide, and he enters from between them.
   c. A variation of girl on top: He lies on his back and draws his knees up to his chest. You can either squat or kneel on either side of his hips and slide onto his cock.
   d. A position where you kneel facing each other: You spread your legs and he thrusts up into you.

8. **What type of lubrication is safe to use when giving him a hand job?**
   a. Water-based lube
   b. Warming lube
   c. Silicone-based lube
   d. Petroleum oil-based lube
   e. Both A and C
   f. All of the above

9. **Why do men have nipples?**
   a. To give you something to hold on to while in the Cowgirl position
   b. To nurse their young should women become extinct
   c. Because nipples are not sex-specific characteristics (as vaginas and penises are)
   d. To enhance the appearance of their chests and attract potential mates

10. **What is the purpose of the foreskin?**
    a. It really has no purpose; it's an extra flap of unnecessary skin on his penis.
    b. It protects the head of his penis.
    c. It makes hand jobs and intercourse smoother and easier.
    d. It creates natural lubrication during sex.
    e. Answers B, C, and D

11. **What is phallophilia?**
    a. A sex position in which you support yourself in a door frame and he takes you from behind
    b. The fear of large penises
    c. The act of giving fellatio while on your grandmother's futon
    d. An obsession with large penises

12. **In ancient Greece, how did athletes keep their penises from flopping in the wind?**
    a. They pierced their foreskin and attached it to a second piercing on the scrotum.
    b. They wore jock straps made from sheep's wool.
    c. They tied their foreskin to the base of their penis with a thin leather ribbon.
    d. They wore "tighty whities" made from lion skin.
    e. They wore nothing, which is where the phrase "going commando" comes from.

13. **What is penis panic?**
    a. A funny way to describe erectile dysfunction (when a guy can't get it up)
    b. A mass cultural belief that penises are slowly retracting and will eventually disappear
    c. A funny way to describe premature ejaculation (when a man ejaculates too quickly)
    d. The feeling a guy gets after he's been struck in the testicles

14. **What part of a woman's body do the majority of men like to look at during sex?**
    a. Your face
    b. Your breasts
    c. Your legs
    d. Your ass
    e. Your lasagna

15. **What can cause erectile dysfunction?**
    a. Diseases such as diabetes and heart disease
    b. Smoking, drinking, or doing drugs
    c. Going to Catholic school
    d. Lack of sleep caused by the pitter-patter of little feet
    e. All of the above

16. **What are Kegels?**
    a. A sex position that resembles doing a keg stand, only instead of sucking on a keg nozzle, you suck on his penis
    b. An exercise in which he squeezes his pelvic floor, giving him better bladder control (and potentially making him a better lover)
    c. An exercise that works to tighten his scrotum so that it doesn't hang too low as he ages
    d. The scientific term to describe the orgasmic contractions that precede ejaculation

17. **How frequently should a man ejaculate?**
    a. No more than once per month—too frequent ejaculation can cause problems such as heart disease, priapism, and epilepsy
    b. No more than once per week, especially if he's trying to get you pregnant—we don't want to use all of his baby makers up.
    c. As frequently as he likes—ejaculating may even prevent prostate cancer.
    d. Daily to avoid DSB (deadly sperm buildup)

18. **What is the evolutionary purpose of the corona?**
    a. To provide the relaxing effects of alcohol that lead to uninhibited sex and better chances of reproduction
    b. To scrape other men's semen from the vagina, thereby increasing a man's chances of reproduction
    c. To increase a woman's pleasure, leading her to seek penises with wider coronas; this, in turn, gives the bearer more chances to reproduce.
    d. To provide an extra holding cell for sperm; when a man finally has sex he ejaculates more, thereby increasing his chances of reproduction.

19. **What is the meatus?**
    a. The scientific word for the (meaty) penile shaft
    b. The sensitive spot on the underside of his cock, where the head meets the shaft
    c. The opening of the urethra where semen and urine pass through
    d. The small strip of skin between his legs, located just between his rectum and his scrotum (otherwise known as the taint)
    e. A term used to describe a highschool bully

20. **How many sperm can be found in a teaspoon of semen?**
    a. 14 to 80, depending on the age of the man
    b. 2 to 5,000
    c. 2 million to 5 million
    d. 200 to 500 million
    e. 1 billion or more

PENIS IQ RESULTS

- If you answered **0 to 4** questions correctly, you are a penis novice.

- If you answered **5 to 9** questions correctly, you are a penis student.

- If you answered **10 to 14** questions correctly, you are a penis professional.

- If you answered **15 to 19** questions correctly, you are a penis scholar.

- If you answered **20 of 20** questions correctly, congratulations! **You are a penis genius!**

 MY PENIS IQ SCORE:

 # PENIS IQ ANSWERS

1. d	8. f	15. e
2. b	9. c	16. b
3. a	10. e	17. c
4. d	11. d	18. b
5. e	12. c	19. c
6. e	13. b	20. d
7. c	14. a	

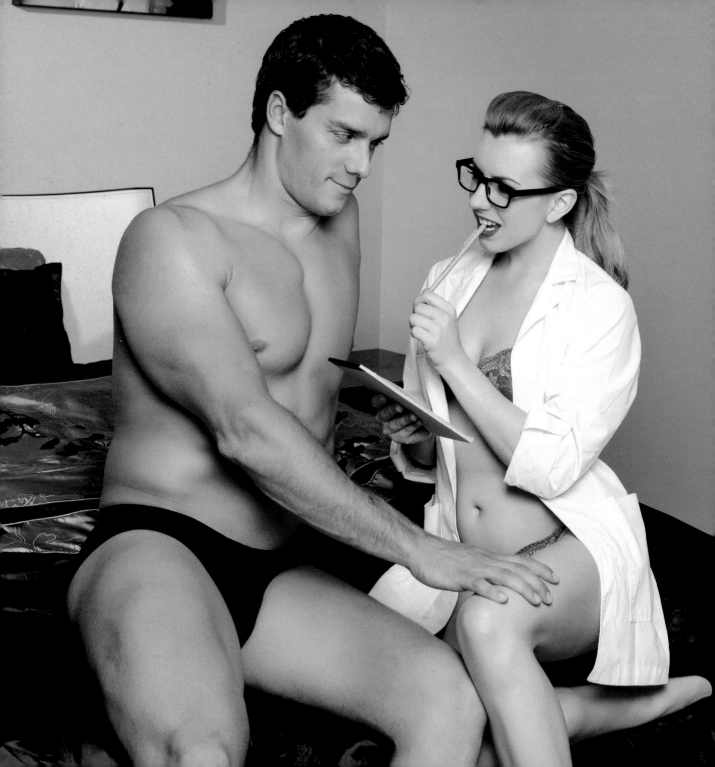

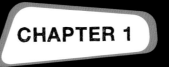

CHAPTER 1

PENIS ANATOMY: A PLEASURE ROAD MAP

You may have seen a detailed illustration of penis anatomy at your doctor's office, but this lesson is unlike any your M.D. would ever give you. From corona to shaft, from frenulum to scrotum, we'll give you a step-by-step road map of his pleasure stick, and along the way we'll let you know which parts are most responsive to sexual stimulation and how to expertly handle them. We'll also let you know which areas to be careful around. (The meatus, for example, is extremely sensitive to alcohol; this is one case where meat and wine don't mix!)

LAB WORK - TAKE A TOUR

Purpose:
To determine how different areas of your guy's penis respond to a variety of tactile sensations

What you'll need:
Warming lube, a glass of ice cubes, a lab notebook and pencil, white lab coat (lingerie optional), sexy spectacles, and high heels

The method:

❶ Surprise your lover in the middle of his day with a dirty phone call. Notify him that your favorite plaything, his penis, will be needed for a scientific experiment of the utmost importance. Tell him you expect him to be nude, ready, and waiting at 8 p.m. sharp. Location: the bedroom.

❷ Using the road map provided in this chapter, examine the various parts of his pecker (e.g., shaft, glans penis, frenulum). Locate each zone and become familiar with it.

❸ Try the following sensory experiments on each specific part. For best results, allow him to reset between each experiment–ideally, he will completely relax and return to a flaccid state. This may require spreading the experiment out over the course of a few hours (or days). If at any point he ejaculates, be sure to give him plenty of time to get back to the very beginning stages of arousal before moving on to the next experiment.

❹ Use just your dry fingers to caress each part.

❺ Use your tongue to lick each part.

❻ Use an ice cube to stimulate each part.

❼ Use a warming lube and massage it into each part.

❽ Ask your guy to describe in detail how your touch feels. Note his responses. Also write down in your lab notebook any discernible nonverbal reactions he gives you (e.g., Does he moan, laugh, scream, or sigh? Does his cock harden or soften? Do his testicles tighten?).

Optional: Illustrate your own personal map of his male anatomy.

The conclusion:
After you've concluded this specific experiment, you'll be far more aware of the pleasure points on your man's penis and will have a handle on how to best manhandle him for mutual satisfaction. But don't let the experimenting end here! Ask him if there are any other tactile sensations he might be curious about. (For example, would he like to donate his cock to the study of ticklers or vibrating toys?) The more you experiment, the more you'll be able to truly understand your man's likes and dislikes. Use the information you gather from these experiments to truly master your man's penis pleasure.

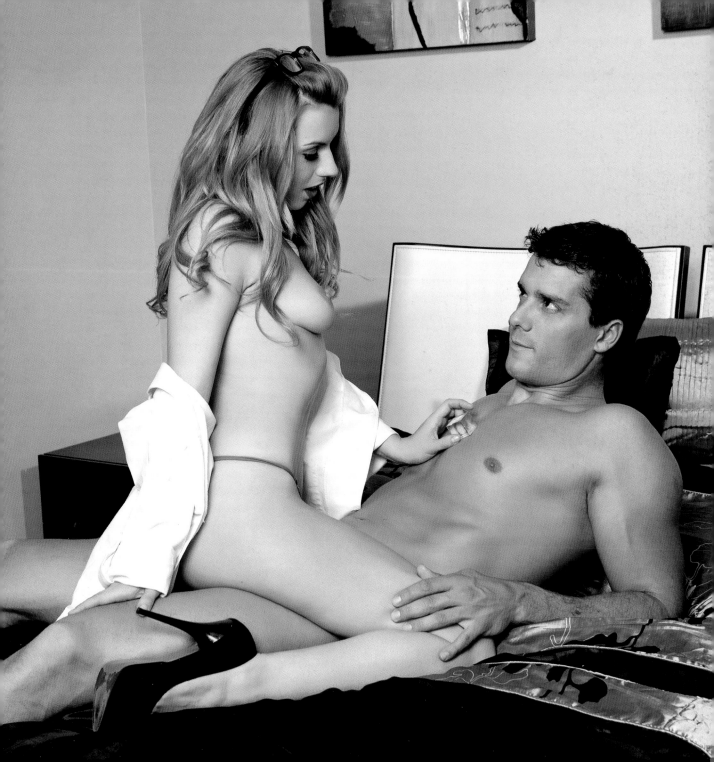

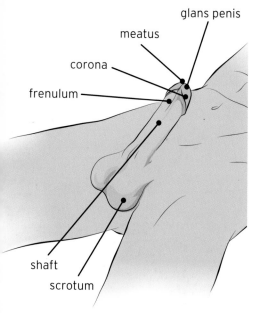

glans penis
meatus
corona
frenulum
shaft
scrotum

PENIS SHAFT

Where to Find It

The penis shaft is that shape-shifting pillar of flesh that sometimes (or quite often when in your sexy presence) juts out from between his legs. When flaccid (due to cold temperatures, anxiety, mundane activities, and surprise visits from your mother), it does a lot less jutting and hangs freely between his legs. It might appear shriveled and loose, or completely bundled up like a turtle in its shell.

Its Purpose

Without a shaft, there would be nothing to erect for his erection. The shaft contains three columns of spongy erectile tissue; two are called *corpora cavernosa*, and the third, which wraps around the urethra, is the *corpora spongiosum*. The tissue is interlaced by a network of arteries that, when aroused, fill up with blood, creating a sight that most women are very familiar with: the raging hard-on. After ejaculation, dorsal veins drain the blood out of his penis (and hopefully send it back to his brain).[1]

Indications

As the largest area of his penis, his shaft offers a ton of fun to be had. Wrap your hands around it and stroke, wrap your lips around it and lick and suck, wrap your breasts around it and titty-fuck, and of course wrap your legs around it and ride. Says Colin, a thirtysomething doctoral student, "I love fast little licks on the underside of my shaft—delivered sideways, instead of up and down."

The base of the shaft begins inside his body, underneath the testicles. You can access this part of his shaft by pressing your forefinger or hand, lengthwise, to the center of his scrotum. Use slow, careful pressure to separate the testicles. Gently rub back and forth until you get to the base of the scrotum, where you will indirectly make contact with the hidden bottom of his shaft. If he likes it, continue the massage.

Much like the interior of your vaginal canal (as opposed to your labia and clitoris), the shaft of your man's penis is very responsive to pressure.

Stimulating the head of his cock and surrounding areas with your tongue while keeping a firm or pulsating grip on his shaft may be just what the doctor ordered.

Contraindications

It's hard to go wrong with the shaft, but unless your guy is into penile pain, don't bite, don't pull on it like a tug rope, and *please* don't give him any Indian rug burns.

GLANS PENIS

Where to Find It

Glans penis is the scientific word for his little head (as opposed to his big head, which is where he presumably keeps his brain). It's the helmet that sits atop the shaft, and it houses a great number of nerve endings.

Its Purpose

Among other unusual attributes—like fully opposable thumbs, an inexplicable love for televised sports, and (compared to other primates) relatively hair-free skin—human males are the only species who have a little head below their belts. This has caused scientists to wonder about the evolutionary purpose of this bulbous addition to his shaft. The unique mushroom shape, aside from being integral to your pleasure, has been postulated to serve an important evolutionary purpose that increases a man's potential for creating offspring. Read more about this hypothesis on page 26.

Indications

Second only to the frenulum, 26 percent of our male survey takers reported that stimulation of the penis head was the most . . . um . . . stimulating. Because of the high concentration of nerve endings and the consequent pleasure principle, the glans penis has been compared to the highly sensitive clitoris. In fact, the two develop from the same tissue in the womb.[3] Now that you can empathize with this particular sensitive spot, you understand the importance of lavishing it with attention. Try licking it

IN OTHER WORDS: FUN VERNACULAR FOR THE PENIS

cock, dick, Johnson, love stick, magic stick, one-eyed Willy, package, pecker, Peter, pickle, pleasure pole, prick, rod, sausage, schlong, tally whacker, tool, unit, wang, wiener (try saying that three times fast!)

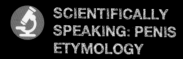
like an ice cream cone and use generous flicks of your tongue. Suck it like a lollipop, or treat it like a pleasurable frosting spatula by taking his shaft in your hand and using the glans to spread the juices of your slick vaginal lips or to stimulate your clit. Says Leo, a twentysomething actor, "My most sensitive spot is my head. I love it when my partner licks it or just sucks the head. I also love to squeeze my head when I'm jacking off."

Contraindications

Use common sense. Just as you wouldn't want him to rub your clit raw, treat him the same by keeping your touch slippery and soft.

CORONA

Where to Find It

No, we're not talking about a refreshing bottle of beer garnished with a slice of lime. Corona is Spanish for *crown*, and it describes that little ridge of flesh that separates the head of his cock from the shaft.

Its Purpose

Some scientists conjecture that the corona (or coronal ridge), aside from making his penis look like royalty, also serves as a semen displacement device. In 2003, a team of psychologists led by Gordon Gallup and Rebecca Burch from the State University of New York risked being shunned at university functions by undertaking a quirky study of this odd little piece of anatomy. They hypothesized that the corona is shaped specifically so that it can scrape other men's semen out of a woman's vaginal canal, by way of vigorous thrusting. The purpose is to eliminate genetic competition.

To test this hypothesis, the team used a fake pussy, of the type found at your local sex store, and three dildos, one with a large coronal ridge, another with a smaller ridge, and a third without any ridge at all. Instead of collecting bucketfuls of real semen from horny university students, they (wisely) made a concoction of unbleached flour and water to replicate the real stuff. They filled the fake vagina with the goo and then, using each phallus in turn, recreated a thrusting motion, similar to the one your guy treats you to during a hot round of coitus. The result? Both dildos with the coronal ridges displaced 91 percent of the semen, while the headless toy only displaced 35 percent of the gunk. They also found that the deeper the thrust, the more semen was displaced.[4,5]

Think about the possible implications of this study! It could indicate that men have evolved to compete for reproduction rights with women who are, by nature, not monogamous. This could support the idea that humans are not wired for monogamy at all. (Oh behave, you little trollops!)

Indications

As a part of his glans, the flesh around the corona is very sensitive to pleasure. Says Dave, a teacher, forty-four, "My sensitive spot is the top of my glans along the ridge. I like it being licked or gently rubbed with a lubricated thumb."

Contraindications

With sensitivity to pleasure comes sensitivity to pain. Handle with care.

FRENULUM

Where to Find It

Everyone has several frenula on their body; find one of yours by licking along the upper front side of your gums where they meet the inside of your upper lip. Feel that taught membrane? That is a frenulum. Your guy just so happens to have one on the underside of his penis where the glans and shaft connect.

Its Purpose

On uncircumcised men, the frenulum helps the foreskin slide back and forth over the glans. On circumcised men, this little piece of his penis has nothing to support or restrain, so it serves more as a pleasure spot than anything else.

In our survey, 41% of men said their frenulum is the most sensitive spot on their cocks. Lightly caress and lick this area during sex play. Try massaging the area with your thumb using soft, circular motions, while caressing his glans with the rest of your fingers.

SCIENTIFICALLY SPEAKING: WHAT IS A FRENULUM?

The general definition for *frenulum* is a small fold of tissue that prevents an organ in the body from moving too far, or a connecting fold of membrane to support or restrain a part.[8] There are several frenula in the mouth, some in the digestive tract, and women also have frenula connected to the external genitalia, including one attaching to the clitoris.[9]

Indications

In our survey, 41 percent of men said their frenulum is the most sensitive spot on their cocks. Lightly caress and lick this area during sex play. Try massaging the area with your thumb using soft, circular motions, while caressing his glans with the rest of your fingers.

If you are eager for your guy to ejaculate, a rhythmic stroking of this particular spot could do the trick. Says Jacob, a fiftysomething writer, "There is nothing better than a long, slow finger-rub on the frenulum (using cocoa butter lube). It is a strokeless way of masturbating. Who knew you could do it with one finger? It can take ten minutes and results in an outstanding orgasm—although it doesn't work unless I haven't come for several days."

Says Will, a fiftysomething truck driver, "The spot under the head, the frenulum, is probably the most sensitive spot on my entire body . . . especially after I come. My loving wife loves to lick it . . . trying to send me through the headboard!"

Contraindications

Some uncircumcised men may have a condition called *frenulum breve*, which is a shortened frenulum. For these guys, it's difficult for the foreskin to pull back completely from the glans, and it can cause painful sex or even little tears in the sensitive flesh. Men with this condition are often told that the only solution is circumcision. However, there is another, less invasive procedure called frenuloplasty, a ten-minute outpatient method that loosens the frenulum so that the foreskin can properly retract.[10]

FORESKIN

Where to Find It

In the United States, it may be difficult to find the foreskin. (We are a foreskin-challenged nation!) According to the U.S. Department of Health and Human Services, currently 60 percent of American males had their foreskins removed via circumcision in infancy (down from 85 percent for those babies born in the 1970s).[11] However, if you have the opportunity to encounter an intact penis, you can recognize the foreskin as that skin resembling a cozy little sleeping bag that covers the head of his penis when it's flaccid. When erect, the glans comes out from its shell, and the foreskin appears more like a bunched up sock just beneath the head. Foreskin is very elastic and mobile, and can be a source of great pleasure for you both.

Its Purpose
The foreskin (also known as the prepuce) has many purposes. Among other functions, it protects his glans from irritation and chafing, creates natural lubrication during masturbation and sex, facilitates penetration during sex (the unfolding foreskin allows the penis to enter the vagina without friction, eliminating the need to "force" it in), and contains a high density of nerve endings that enhance his pleasure.[12] (Read more about the foreskin in chapter five.)

Indications
When giving a hand job or blow job, don't neglect this erogenous zone. Try moving the elastic flesh of the foreskin up and down over his glans. The area just inside the tip of his foreskin is particularly sensitive to pleasure—try gently massaging the inside, or flick your tongue under the skin and around the "lips" of the foreskin (where it opens for the glans). Says Rick, a sixtysomething retired structural engineer, "I love it when a woman pushes my foreskin back with her tongue."

Contraindications
The biggest concern with intact men is cleanliness. Small glands beneath the foreskin produce a cheesy, stinky substance called smegma. To avoid irritation and infection, it's important for men to keep their parts clean and tidy and not allow the substance to build up. Nothing can ruin a blow job faster than the overpowering scent of Camembert in his shorts.[13]

FAMOUS PENIS: DAVID

Think you've never seen an uncircumcised penis? Think again. Look closely at Michelangelo's famous statue of David. You'll notice that he sports a stonier version of a flaccid, uncut penis.

MEATUS

Where to Find It

The meatus is the little slit at the top of his glans.

Its Purpose

No, the meatus isn't the eye of the one-eyed wonder worm! It's the opening of the urethra, where both urine and semen exit the penis.

Indications

Using either a lubricated palm or finger, or your tongue, you can gently massage or lick the opening. Sensitive mucous membranes around the opening can be susceptible to pleasure if touched wetly and lightly. Says Chris, a thirty-three-year-old financial adviser, "I love to have my slit gently licked during a blow job, but I'd prefer her to use her fingers elsewhere, as a wrong move here can really hurt."

Contraindications

These sensitive mucous membranes can be easily irritated. A lot of men would prefer you not to tread too closely to this spot, so be careful. If your guy is open to a little meatus stimulation, never use a dry hand around this area because it can cause the slit to uncomfortably pull open and you can even accidentally scrape him.

It's best not to introduce irritating substances such as alcohol or hot chili peppers to the meatus. As romantic as it sounds to take a mouthful of Pinot Noir and go down on your partner, don't! The alcohol in the wine can sting when it comes in contact with that tiny opening, just like rubbing alcohol stings when you rub it on a cut. Other spicy or acidic foods may have the same effect. So unless your guy is into pain, try a cool glass of water instead.

Note that sexually transmitted infections can be passed through this opening. Use condoms, and keep your mouth away if you have sores or cuts.[14] (For more information on STIs, see chapter nine.)

SCROTUM

Where to Find It

The scrotum is that oft-ignored sack of flesh containing his testicles that hangs below your man's penis.

Its Purpose

The main function is to keep the testicles at the optimum temperature for generating sperm. While the rest of the body is comfortable at 98.6°F (37°C), the testes prefer a cooler temperature of 93°F (34°C), keeping the little swimmers at the ready for action. When things get a little too cold for comfort outside, the scrotum wrinkles and tightens, hugging the testicles close to the body for added warmth.[15]

Indications

Although it may not look as beautiful as your guy's penis, the scrotum is a powerhouse of pleasure. Try gently tugging down on his sack as you give him a blow job. During a hand job, try very gently sucking first one testicle and then the other into your mouth. Says Tyler, a thirty-seven-year-old evolutionary geneticist, "A woman who plays with my balls is priceless. I love to have them grabbed, rubbed, licked, sucked, etc." To give him a real sensory treat, lick or caress the line that runs down the center of his scrotum. This little treasure trail is called the scrotal raphe, pronounced *RAY-fee*.

Contraindications

Don't be too rough with his family jewels. Since the scrotum contains the very sensitive testes, avoid jabbing, hitting, or knocking these guys together. For men, getting hit in the nuts is one of the most painful things to endure. (Lucky guys—they never have to deal with menstrual cramps or childbirth.) Take heart and spare him the pain so he can trust you with his fun little playthings.

Once you have your guy's penis mapped out, it's time for a sexy expedition. Travel, explore, and enjoy his unique hot spots. He'll be dubbing you a penis genius before you know it!

IN OTHER WORDS: FUN VERNACULAR FOR THE TESTICLES

bag, balls, ball sack, the boys, coin purse, cojones, the downunders, family jewels, figs, gonads, the homies, juevos, kiwis, lefticle and righticle, low hangers, nads, nuts, nut sack, plums, rocks, sperm dorm, the step-children, stones, tea bag, the twins, yogurt factory

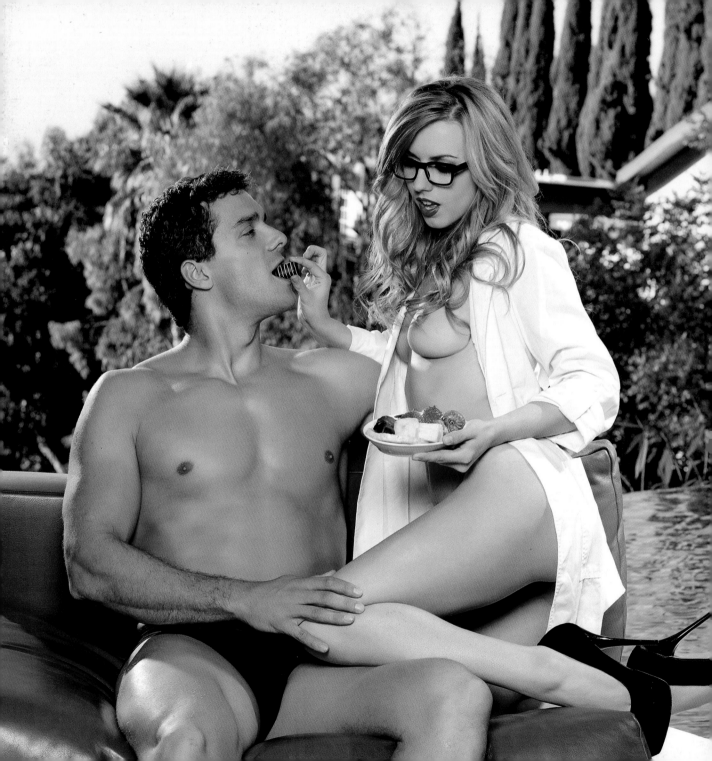

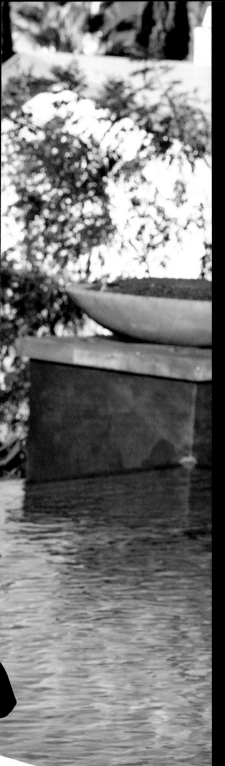

CHAPTER 2

HIS SPECIAL SAUCE: ALL THE FLAVORS OF HIS PUDDING

Ejaculation is the final show in a man's typical sexual encounter. From the money-shot so often and openly displayed in porn, to his final grunts and spasms during coitus, the eruption of semen can be compared to the fireworks finale at a New Year's Eve party. As such, the mysterious substance lends itself to a variety of questions, concerns, and lore.

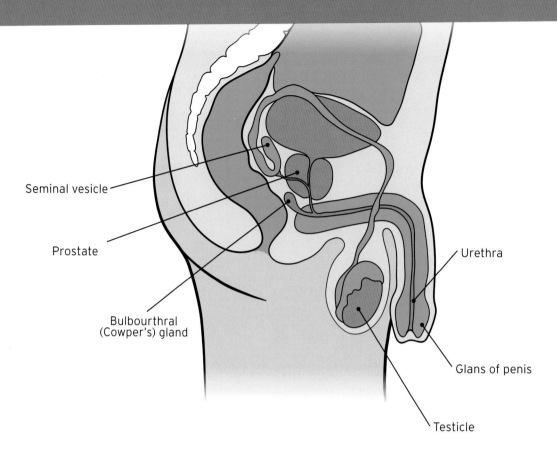

Seminal vesicle

Prostate

Bulbourthral
(Cowper's) gland

Urethra

Glans of penis

Testicle

For starters, let's get the facts straight about the difference between semen and sperm. Semen is the sticky fluid that erupts from your guy's penis when you bring him to orgasm. Usually, he'll shoot about a teaspoon of the stuff for each ejaculation. The seminal fluid carries the little baby makers known as spermatozoa, or sperm. There are approximately 200 million to 500 million sperm in each ejaculation, but they are so tiny that they only make up about 1 percent of the total concoction.

There are a lot of cooks in the semen kitchen. The testicles are responsible for producing the actual sperm, but only about 5 percent of the total seminal fluid. The rest of the brew is produced by various glands in your guy's body. The seminal vesicles, for example, produce the seminal plasma—think of this as the thickening base ingredient in your man's soup—which makes up about 45 percent to 80 percent of the total fluid. The prostate gland contributes 15 percent to 30 percent of semen's volume in the form of prostate fluid, which we like to think of as a flavorful preservative. This milky, alkaline fluid neutralizes the acidity in a woman's vagina and uterus, helping to protect the sperm as they make the arduous trek toward the egg. Other glands providing smaller amounts of seasoning to the tasty concoction include the bulbourethral (Cowper's) and urethral glands.[16]

PRESENTATION OF THE SEMEN SOUP

Now that we have a basic understanding of the recipe for ejaculate, let's talk about its plating and presentation. The delivery of semen is a pointedly interactive experience for both parties, and because of this, you and your lover may have an array of questions about its color, consistency, taste, potency, and even the amount that comes out.

Why Is Some Cum Watery While Other Spooge Is Creamy?

If real life were like the porn industry, all men would shoot spurt after spurt of creamy, milky white semen. In reality, semen varies in color, quantity, and consistency from man to man and even from orgasm to orgasm. The variation is due to a number of factors, including how much water your man has been drinking (more water can help produce more semen) and how many times he's ejaculated in a specific time span (if he's not given time to build up his reserves, the amount of cum will decrease with each shot).[17] It's normal for semen to be white, yellowish, or even grey in color. Note: Pink semen may indicate the presence of blood, and if it persists, he should seek medical attention.

If your guy doesn't ejaculate at all when he orgasms, he's likely experiencing retrograde ejaculation, where the semen goes backward in his urethra down to the bladder instead of shooting out the meatus. Retrograde ejaculation is rare and, in and of itself, is not a major health concern unless you're trying to get pregnant. However, retrograde ejaculation can be a side effect of certain high blood pressure and

Many men seem to be concerned with producing a nice, healthy helping of baby batter, whether or not they're actually trying to make a baby. Some men may correlate a large helping to impressive sexual prowess.

mood-altering medications, surgery, or diabetes, in which cases your man should consult with his physician to manage the cause.[18]

Is It Possible to Increase the Volume of Ejaculate?

Many men seem to be concerned with producing a nice, healthy helping of baby batter, whether or not they're actually trying to make a baby. Some men may correlate a large helping to impressive sexual prowess. There is a small amount of biology behind the desire for an increased volume of semen. A larger amount means more sperm (and thus a greater chance of impregnation), as well as more or stronger muscle contractions required to spurt the stuff out (and thus more pleasurable orgasms).

Unfortunately, there's not a lot of hard science to inform us on how to increase seminal volume. Some sex experts recommend amino acids such as L-arginine and L-lysine, zinc, as well as Horny Goat Weed plant. Increasing fluids is another suggestion. And abstaining from coming for a day or two (rather than an hour or two) will ensure optimum semen levels.[19]

How Far Should Semen Shoot?

In their breakthrough book *Human Sexual Response*, doctors William H. Masters and Virginia E. Johnson report that when unhindered, the first contraction of a male ejaculation can propel his semen one to two feet (0.3 to 0.6 meters).[20] However, some men may experience only a small dribble of ejaculate upon orgasm. Both scenarios are normal, and neither are cause for concern. Internet lore reports that a man named Horst Schultz achieved an ejaculation that shot 18 feet, 9 inches at 42.7 miles per hour (about 5.7 meters at 68.7 km/hour).[21] Even if this is possible, unless your guy is a secret agent and needs to be able to use his penis as a weapon, what's the point? During sex, his cock is typically inside some orifice of your body or contained in a condom, and the actual distance he can ejaculate is null.

What Semens to Be the Problem?

It's all naughty fun and games until someone gets semen in the eye. If this happens to you, don't panic! The stuff stings about as much as a dollop of shampoo and it's as easily treated. Simply rinse your eye out with cool water.

There is a small chance that you can contract an STI from semen-to-eye contact (especially diseases such as chlamydia and gonorrhea),[22] so watch for any rashes or sores that may develop, especially if you're not sure about the health of your sex partner. In the future, close your eyes tightly when he shoots his load in the direction of your chest or face, or if you're up for a little sexy scientist role-playing, wear lab goggles!

TIPS ON MAKING CUM TASTE BETTER

Scientists haven't yet undertaken an experiment to determine whether diet affects the flavor of his semen, although most people believe it does. (This holds true for women's lubrications, too!) We suppose a laboratory-style test of this hypothesis could pose some serious challenges. Ultimately, it's up to you to experiment on your own and decide whether pineapple (or anything else) truly makes his pudding taste sweeter.

If you are the type of girl who likes to swallow but sometimes gets offended by the flavor of his spunk, here are a few fun ways to take the ick out of his love stick.

Shoot It Like Tequila, or an Oyster!

Just because you swallow doesn't mean you have to swish the stuff around in your mouth like you would a mouthful of fine Malbec. When he ejaculates, simply push the head of his cock past your taste buds toward the back of your throat and swallow it down. No muss, no fuss.

Add Your Own Flavor

Try sucking on a lollipop or a mint before (or even during) a blow job, or coat his shaft (avoiding his meatus) with a powdered candy such as Pop Rocks or Fun Dips. But don't use mouthwash, chili peppers, or lemons, as these can irritate his penis, and don't chew gum during a blow job, or you'll run the risk of accidentally chomping down on him! As a safe but not necessarily as tasty alternative, try one of the many varieties of flavored lubrication and powders available at sex toy stores.

IN OTHER WORDS: FUN VERNACULAR FOR EJACULATE

cum, frosting, baby batter, baby gravy, busting a nut, the explosion at the yogurt factory, goo, jizz, liquid gold, love cream, magic sauce, money shot, penis pudding, population paste, shooting his wad, special sauce, spooge, spunk, wonder worms

LAB WORK - TASTE TEST

Purpose:
To determine whether diet can change the flavor of your man's semen

What you'll need:
Pineapple, asparagus, chocolate, coffee, lab notebook, pencil, white lab coat (lingerie optional), sexy spectacles, high heels

The method:

1 Take your lover grocery shopping and hand him a shopping list titled "Blow Job Foods." The list should include each of the foods you plan to experiment with and the date of the expected blow job. Nonchalantly explain the rules of the taste test experiment as you go about the mundane task of picking up groceries together. (This kind of sexual tease in an everyday place can serve as excellent foreplay.)

2 This experiment will take place over the course of three weeks and will include five blow jobs. To fully participate, you must taste and swallow his special sauce. Note that if your man has issue with any of the test foods, you may substitute the item for

something else—for example, bananas can be substituted for pineapple, alcohol for coffee, red meat for asparagus, and ice cream for chocolate. For best results, aside from the test foods, your man should eat a consistent diet throughout the experiment with little to no variation. Keep track of everything he eats each day in your lab journal.

DAY ONE: Begin with your control blow job. Before introducing any of the test foods to his diet, give your guy some knockout oral sex (see chapter three for tips on giving great head). Write down a detailed description of the flavor of his semen: Does he taste sweet like candy? Salty like French fries? Pungent like an aged cheese? Bitter like Campari?

DAYS TWO THROUGH SIX: The pineapple test. Your guy must eat two cups of pineapple every day, while avoiding chocolate, asparagus, and coffee. On day six, give him his second blow job. Again, write down a detailed description of the flavor of his semen.

DAYS SEVEN THROUGH ELEVEN: The coffee test. Your guy must drink two cups of coffee every day, while avoiding pineapple, chocolate, and asparagus. On day eleven, give him his third blow job. Again, write down a detailed description of the flavor of his semen.

DAYS TWELVE THROUGH SIXTEEN: The chocolate test. Your guy must eat four ounces (113 grams) of chocolate every day, while avoiding pineapple, coffee, and asparagus. On day sixteen, give him his fourth blow job. Again, write down a detailed description of the flavor of his semen.

DAYS SEVENTEEN THROUGH TWENTY-ONE: The asparagus test. Your guy must eat one cup of asparagus every day, while avoiding pineapple, chocolate, and coffee. On day twenty-one, give him his fifth blow job. Again, write down a detailed description of the flavor of his semen.

EVALUATE YOUR NOTES.

Did the flavor of his semen change over time? How did the flavor correspond to each of the test foods? Did it taste sweeter? Saltier? More bitter? Or did the flavor remain constant?

Optional: Continue the experiment and try adding or eliminating the following substances to or from his diet: alcohol, red meat, and soda.

The conclusion:

You might discover that adding or removing certain foods from his diet will make giving him a blow job that much more pleasurable for you. What fun it would be for both of you to find a magic combination that would make you crave the flavor of his cock even more!

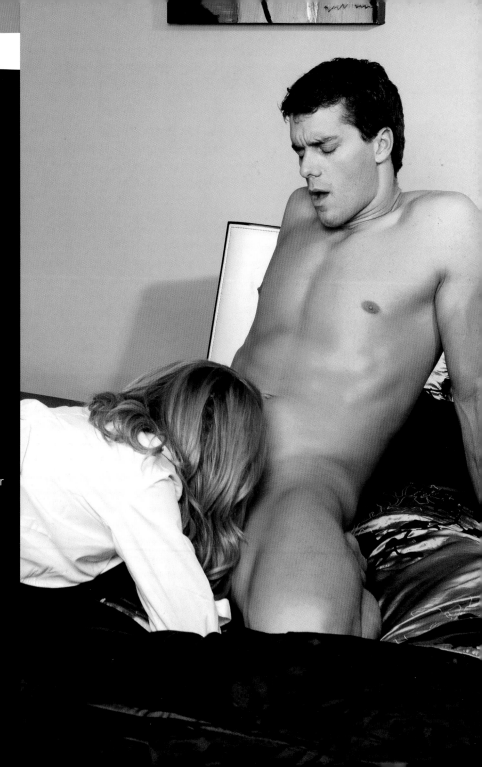

Once you've been with your partner for some time, you should become accustomed to and perhaps even enjoy the way he tastes. Think of his semen as being like sophisticated hors d'oeuvres at a fancy French restaurant; it's an acquired taste.

Taste Is in the Nose

If you've ever had a stuffy nose, you know the effect that your sense of smell has on your taste buds. Try experimenting with this interaction by placing a drop of perfume on your upper lip, or filling the room with scented candles or the scent of homemade cinnamon rolls. You may find that the pleasing smells filling your nose will make his cum shot that much more palatable. You can also try to not breathe through your nose when you swallow, but we don't advise you wear an unseemly looking nose plug or pinch your nose with your fingers while you are going down on him.

An Acquired Taste

Once you've been with your partner for some time, you should become accustomed to and perhaps even enjoy the way he tastes. Think of his semen as being like sophisticated hors d'oeuvres at a fancy French restaurant; it's an acquired taste.

THE PRACTICAL SIDE OF SEMEN: CONCEPTION

Indeed, it is fun to squirt his juice on your boobs, or surprise him by swallowing it down like a naughty girl. But the ultimate purpose of semen is to produce itty-bitty babies that turn into cute kids, and then evil teens, and eventually, responsible, well-rounded adults who could someday be president.

Out of the millions of sperm in each glorious ejaculation, it only takes one victorious swimmer to conceive; however, sometimes finding that singular little guy is a challenge (unless of course you are *not* trying to get pregnant, which miraculously makes getting knocked up as easy as ordering pizza). If you are looking to conceive, here are some important tips to help make sure that your guy's magic sauce is in tip-top baby-making shape.

Limit His Time in the Hot Tub

There is a reason that his scrotum keeps such careful tabs on the temperature of his testicles. If his nuts get too hot (98°F/37°C or warmer), they turn into lazy good-for-nothings and put a halt on sperm production. Spending thirty minutes or more in a hot tub can lower his sperm count for months, since it takes about three months for his body to produce these wonder worms. Note that this rule only pertains to direct heat applied to his crotch.[23]

Avoid Drinking Alcohol and Smoking Cigarettes

Researchers in the Department of Pathology at the Himalayan Institute of Medical Sciences found that both alcohol and cigarettes negatively impact male fertility. The scientists compared the sperm of one hundred alcoholics and one hundred smokers with that of one hundred nonsmoking, nondrinking good boys. They found that alcoholics suffered a low sperm count (referred to as oligozoospermia). The drinkers also produced a lot of abnormal-looking sperm, scientifically known as teratozoospermia (*terato* means monster, so you could call it "monster sperm"), as opposed to their nondrinking counterparts. While the study found that smokers produced a normal quantity of sperm, many of them were deformed monster sperm. Smokers also showed more instances of weak sperm with low motility, which is a condition known as asthenozoospermia (just picture the little guys gasping for breath as they're trying to make the long swim to your golden egg).[24] If you and your honey are serious about getting pregnant, he should lay off of these vices at least until the magic moment happens.

More Sex, Less Masturbation

We don't want to discourage masturbation, as it is a very healthy practice for him in general. However, if he is dealing with low sperm count when you are trying to conceive, it's helpful if he saves his best batches of baby batter for you. This is especially important around the time you are ovulating. Saving up for sex helps improve the quality of his semen by capitalizing on his sperm reserves.[25]

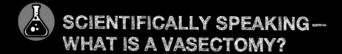

SCIENTIFICALLY SPEAKING— WHAT IS A VASECTOMY?

For those men who are absolutely positive that they don't want to make any (more) babies, a vasectomy is the most reliable (more than 99 percent effective) and permanent method of male birth control. Although getting a vasectomy is painful, and a lot of men may whine and demand ice cream and full control of the remote during recovery, it's not that big of a deal when compared to other surgical procedures. A vasectomy is performed as an outpatient procedure that takes about a half hour at his doctor's office. The doctor starts by giving a local anesthetic to numb his nuts, then pokes two teeny tiny holes in either side of his scrotum to access the vas deferens tubes (the two ducts that sperm travel down on their way out of his testicles). The doctor cuts a small part of these vas deferens and seals the ends shut; the holes are so small that typically your lover won't need stitches. He'll be sent home with instructions to ice his junk, watch sports, and avoid sex for a couple of weeks.

In a few weeks, your guy will need to jack off into a cup for the laboratory to test for sperm. Before he's cleared for baby-free sex, he'll need to generate two consecutive samples of sperm-free semen, which can take three months or more. After all is said and done, he'll still orgasm and ejaculate as he did before—after all, he's now missing only less than 5 percent of his total ejaculatory fluid. Some men even report heightened arousal, likely because they're no longer afraid of getting you knocked up.[28]

Technical Difficulties

Some studies indicate that laptops and cell phones may affect his sperm quality. In 2009, researchers in the Department of Environmental Epidemiology at the Nofer Institute of Occupational Medicine in Lodz, Poland, reported that extended cell phone use—four or more hours per day—may decrease sperm count and motility due to the electromagnetic radiation emitted by the devices. However, they admitted that the studies were small and may not be representative of a larger population.[26]

Additionally, in a 2005 study, researchers in the Department of Urology and General Clinical Research Center at the State University of New York at Stony Brook found that men who use laptops (and place them on their laps) significantly increase their scrotal temperature. Application of direct heat to the testicles is a proven factor in low sperm count, as mentioned earlier. Researchers concluded that repeated exposure of his lap to his laptop could have a negative impact on fertility, particularly of young men who are more apt to use this technology over a period of many years. They also stated that further evaluation is needed.[27]

Other Hurdles

It has also been argued that wearing tight underwear, spending a lot of time riding a bicycle, or even sitting for long stretches of time can decrease fertility, as these activities may increase scrotal temperature. It's best for him not to get his tighty whities in a bundle over these habits, unless he's really having serious fertility issues and his doctor suggests he should swap out his briefs for boxers, his bike for jogging shoes, and his desk job for a construction gig.

SEMEN! HUH-YEAH! WHAT IS IT GOOD FOR?

Besides its obvious purpose for procreation, it seems people are always trying to come up with more uses for semen. You might have heard stories that semen is good for your skin, your hair, and your mood. But are they true?

It has also been argued that wearing tight underwear, spending a lot of time riding a bicycle, or even sitting for long stretches of time can decrease fertility, as these activities may increase scrotal temperature. It's best for him not to get his tighty whities in a bundle over these habits.

Semen Is an Excellent Hair Product

A hilarious scene from the 1998 movie *There's Something About Mary* depicts Ted (Ben Stiller) jacking off before his date with Mary (Cameron Diaz) and shooting so hard that he gets some ejaculate on his ear. When he opens the door for Mary, she thinks that his jizz is hair gel and, much to the chagrin (or glee) of viewers, proceeds to scoop it off his ear and rub it in her pretty, blond locks.

It turns out she's not the only woman who has put semen in her hair. In 2008, the swank Hari's Hair & Beauty salon in London offered a hair treatment that was said to nourish and revitalize the hair. The secret ingredient? Bull semen. For a while it was the trendiest treatment in London, with women paying over $100 to have their hair coated in bovine spooge. The idea was that the protein punch delivered by the semen would make hair stronger and shinier and even help it grow. However, Hari has since taken chilled bull semen off the menu and replaced it with a less offensive keratin and avocado oil treatment.[29,30]

Semen Is Good for Your Skin

Proponents of using semen as a moisturizer argue that the solution contains vitamins and salts (from the urethra) that give you a glowing complexion.[31] An unscientific study conducted by two daring individuals for Viceland.com in 2003 proves that this may not be so. One man, twenty-four-year-old Nick, and one woman, twenty-nine-year-old Lisa, agreed to use semen on one cheek, and their usual moisturizer on the other cheek, for four weeks.

At the end of the experiment Nick reported, "I think that thing about cum being good for your skin is a myth straight men made up so women would suck their dicks more often . . . [Using] the man-made cream was just a pain in the ass."

Lisa's result? "I have no doubt that I will never let cum touch my face again. It created a glaze on my cheek, then a rough patch of dead skin. I hope it doesn't take too long to get it back to normal."[32]

While it can be fun to allow your partner to ejaculate on your boobs in the heat of excitement, don't worry about massaging it into your skin. It's probably best to wipe it off, or hop in a nice steamy shower and wash it off after playtime.

Semen Is an Antidepressant

In 2002, researchers led by Gordon Gallup Jr. in the Department of Psychology at the State University of New York at Albany found that females who had sex without condoms were less depressed than their safer-sex-practicing counterparts. They discovered that "not only were females who were having sex without condoms less depressed, but depressive symptoms and suicide attempts among females who used condoms were proportional to the consistency of condom use." They also said women who don't use condoms become more depressed the longer they waited between sexual encounters.[33]

Whether this is true or not, we think that contracting an STI or having an unwanted pregnancy would be much more depressing than using condoms. It's also important to note that, even though the condom users scored higher than their condom-free counterparts on the Beck Depression Inventory scale, most of them didn't even score high enough to be considered moderately depressed.

Semen Can Double as Your Daily Vitamin

According to sex therapist Dr. Jenni Skyler, a teaspoon of semen contains about five calories and is made up of fructose sugar, water, vitamin C, citric acid, protein, and zinc. She says, "Because the calories are so few, the amount of each ingredient is almost microscopic. So don't worry about packing on the pounds if you swallow a little semen, and certainly don't depend on it for any kind of nutritional enhancement."[34]

In 2008, the swank Hari's Hair & Beauty salon in London offered a hair treatment that was said to nourish and revitalize the hair. The secret ingredient? Bull semen.

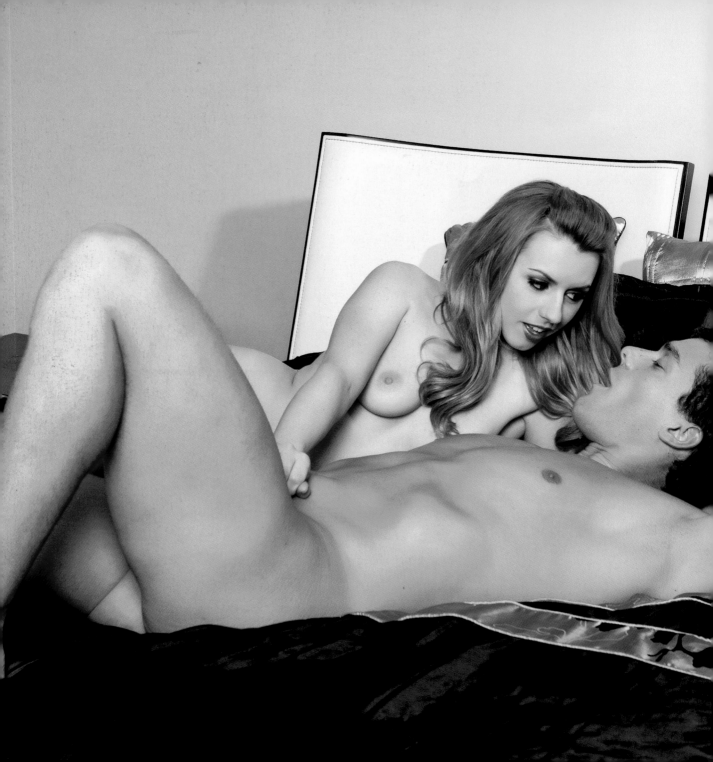

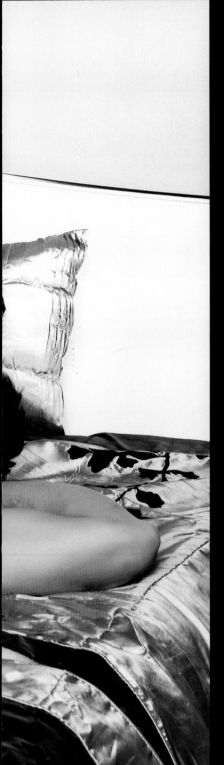

CHAPTER 3

PLAYING WITH DICK: SEXY WAYS TO HANDLE HIS HARD-ON

Now it's time to play with his favorite plaything as if it were yours. Part of becoming a true penis genius is learning and applying exciting, orgasm-inducing techniques. Here are the sexiest ways to handle his hard-on using hand jobs, blow jobs, sex positions, and, yes, even sex toys.

One of the most frequent comments we hear from men regarding blow jobs is, if he can tell you don't like being on the giving end, it's difficult for him to enjoy being on the receiving end.

Before we get started, there are a few ground rules:

❶ Always practice safe sex. Unless you are drug- and disease-free and in a monogamous, long-term relationship, use condoms!

❷ After learning all the tips and tricks in the book, remember that every man is different. What has one man spilling spoonfuls of population pudding onto your bedspread may have another yawning and scratching his nuts. To ensure your sexual success, communicate and find out what your guy wants and needs in the sack.

❸ Remember to ask for his permission, especially when trying new or unusual techniques. If he's never used a cock ring, it would be best to present it to him to inspect before just slipping it over his pecker like a surprise engagement ring. Nothing is worse than being rejected because he's unpleasantly shocked by your explorations.

❹ Keep an open mind and have fun! Sometimes new techniques can induce giggling fits, while others can induce fits of ejaculation. If at first you don't suck-seed, try, try again.

GIVING FANTASTIC FELLATIO

Almost every woman today has given at least a little head in her life. In fact, get a little wine in your best girlfriends, and more than likely you'll have more than a few of them boasting, "I give *the* best blow jobs in the world!" (And more power to the empowered cocksuckers out there!) But whether you're a novice or a connoisseur, there are always a few new signature moves you can put in your oral arsenal.

The Rules
There are a few ground rules to follow when it comes to mouth-on-cock action. Follow these and you're already halfway there to being a great blow job giver:

1. **You have to enjoy it.** One of the most frequent comments we hear from men regarding blow jobs is, if he can tell you don't like being on the giving end, it's difficult for him to enjoy being on the receiving end. Says Dave, a thirty-eight-year-old attorney, "For me to get off during a BJ, she has to enjoy it. If you don't enjoy it, don't waste my time and yours." So unless he has a kink for having you do things you really don't enjoy, approach the blow job as the sexy, playful, and pleasure-giving act it's meant to be. (And for those of you who are reluctant to apply mouth to cock, we offer a few tips later.)

2. **No biting!** Another thing on which men universally agree: Biting is a big no-no when it comes to his penis. So ladies, save the bite marks for his neck.

Tips to Try If the Blow Job Isn't Your Thing (Yet)

If, up to this point, you haven't quite been able to wrap your mind around the joys of giving head, we recommend testing the waters slowly. Here are some things you can try to get your toes wet and make it pleasurable for both of you:

1. **Start in the shower.** Many women are queasy about blow jobs because they're afraid their man isn't clean enough. The solution? Take the cleaning routine into your own hands before you take his cock into your mouth. Washing him gently is also a great way to get him primed for your lip and tongue action. You can even start the sucking right in the shower. Just turn the shower nozzle so you don't get streams of water on your face while you're going down.

2. **Try small licks and soft kisses.** If the thought of taking his entire member into your mouth and sucking like a vacuum is intimidating, start out small with a few tender licks on his cockhead and a trail of sweet kisses down the shaft. When you see how much he enjoys your ministrations, you may be inspired to do a little more each time. You can build your blow job technique in stages and at your own pace.

(continued on page 52)

FROM THE MOUTHS OF OUR TEST SUBJECTS: BLOW JOB POINTERS

When asked what they loved best when getting a blow job, our male survey respondents had some colorful data to contribute:

"Just suck it and slobber all over it— and remember, the operative word is 'job.' She should show up for work wearing boots and a lighted miner's hat." –Jacob, thirty-two, journalist

"Finger in my ass." –Peter, forty-five, professor emeritus

"Patience—and laying her tits in my lap." –Tim, twenty-four, graduate student

And many men reported that there was nothing hotter than having their fellators look them in the eye while going down.

LAB WORK - WHAT'S YOUR FAVORITE PENIS TOPPING?

Purpose:
To match yummy foods and flavors with his natural cock taste

What you'll need:
A sense of adventure, an apron, a well-stocked fridge, a hungry tummy, his penis, a warm and wet washcloth, lab notebook, and pencil

The method:

1 Put on your apron and wear nothing else (except maybe a pair of high heels). Invite your guy into the kitchen. Let him know that you are hungry for a snack, and that the snack you have in mind is *him*.

2 Assemble an assortment of delicious sauces and substances you can lather onto his penis and lick off. Ideas include nonfat whipped cream, strawberry sauce, chocolate sauce, warmed caramel, any of the many flavored lubricants available, melted butter (you can incorporate a small amount of powdered sugar to make this extra decadent), warmed honey, a fruit roll-up (this might necessitate a bit of nibbling on your part), edible body paints, marmalade, and anything else you just love to taste that can be spread on his delectable dick. (Girls, we do warn you to stay away from anything too spicy or acidic, such as hot sauces or picantes. The rule of thumb is, if it burns your tongue, it will burn his cock, too!)

3 Ask him to choose three of the substances.

4 Lay him down and lather him up. Apply one of the things he chose to his cock and lap it off of him with your sexiest kitten licks. Take a moment to note how the substance goes with his personal essence. Then apply the second one and do the same, followed by the third.

5 For best results, take a swallow of cool water to cleanse the palate between each licking session, and keep a warm, wet washcloth and a clean, dry towel on hand for clean-up between flavors.

6 After you've brought him to a delicious climax, ask him which one he liked best. Note it in your lab book.

7 If, after this first round of flavor matching, you haven't quite found the right topping for the perfect blow job, you may have to repeat with other foods or sex aids. You'll just have to tell your man he must sacrifice himself again for the sake of science. Poor baby!

The conclusion:
Just because you find the right flavor combination to top his cock doesn't mean that playtime is over! Have your man reciprocate the experiment as he goes down on you. This exercise is fun foreplay and can lead to more tasty explorations.

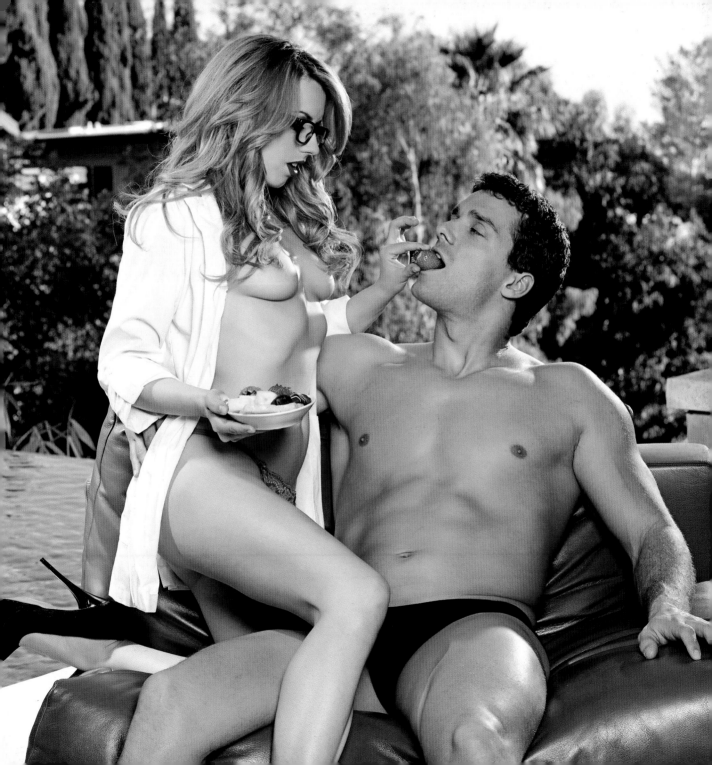

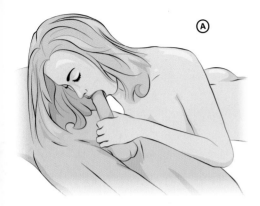

③ **Use the other tools at your disposal.** You don't have to gag yourself to make him feel like he's getting some great head. If you're just not feeling up to using your tongue and mouth to get the whole job done, feel free to use your hands or any other body part to help you out. Swirl your tongue around the head of his cock as you stroke his shaft with your well-lubricated fingers or even a vibrating toy. Remember: The shaft responds to pressure, so while you're sucking his head you can use your hands to simulate the sensations of sex.

Tips to Try If You're Proficient in Penis-Sucking

① **Use your tongue.** It's not all about sucking and swallowing. The tongue is what makes the mouth a unique giver of pleasure. After all, no other body part is equipped with this dexterous little muscle. While giving him a blow job, use it to your advantage!

Try pushing his head into your mouth and leaving your lips loose enough so that you can use your tongue to flick his shaft, alternating from the right, left, and lower sides of his cock. **Ⓐ** Use your tongue like a corkscrew to swirl around his head and upper shaft (watch your teeth when using this technique). You can also use your tongue to stroke his frenulum, the highly sensitive area right under the cockhead on the underside of his penis. **Ⓑ** Or hold the top side of his penis in one hand and lap the underside in long, sensuous licks from his testicles to the tip of his dick and back again. **Ⓒ**

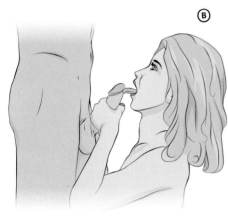

② **Love him with your lips.** Lavish your guy with chaste, angelic kisses. Start at his belly button, kiss down his treasure trail, around his cockhead, down his shaft, and along his testicles. Wear bright red lipstick and leave a trail as you go.

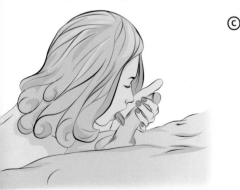

③ **Add a touch of vibration.** When his cock is sliding into your mouth, make long, low, moaning sounds. If you let them reverberate through your throat, they'll add just a touch of a vibrating sensation, which can be quite tantalizing for him. Not to mention that most men love to hear a woman moan–auditory stimulation like this will make the blow job that much hotter.

4 **Tickle with the teeth.** This technique is for the more advanced cocksucker. After all, you have to learn and obey the rules before you can break them. While keeping the "no teeth" rule in mind, be aware that some men enjoy a little bit of toothy stimulation on the shaft—far, far away from the more sensitive head. This is much more of a teeth-tickle than a bite and takes a very light touch.

If your guy is one of these adventurous few, push his cockhead to the back of your mouth and gently graze the skin of his shaft with your teeth. Keep it under control, though; you don't want to accidentally clamp down.

5 **Deep throating.** This "holy grail" move in the world of cocksucking takes some practice, mainly because of that pesky gag reflex. But if you can get your mouth around deep throating, you'll blow him away. True deep throating involves pushing the head of his cock past the uvula (the tear-drop shaped tissue that hangs down at the back of your mouth) and into your throat. While you might not make it this far, even taking his cock in as far as you are able is enough to drive most guys completely out of their minds.

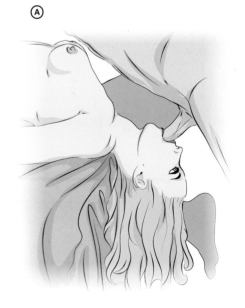

Ⓐ

The key is to relax, get in a position where your neck is extended (lying off the edge of a bed works best Ⓐ), extend your tongue as far as you can, and slowly draw his penis inside as far as you are able. In this position, it will be hard for you to control the sucking motion, so fellatio (sucking) will now become irrumatio (your guy thrusting into your mouth). Stay calm and let him control the motions.

Lubricant is critical, and sometimes saliva just isn't enough. Porn stars use a product called Albolene, which is actually a makeup remover, but it's nontoxic, tasteless, and super-slippery. If you're really serious about deep throat, but you can't get over the gag reflex, you can also try numbing your throat with Chloraseptic spray. Dr. Dick, a clinical sexologist, also reminds us that our gag reflexes are least active in the morning, so this may be a fun way to start your day.

To see deep throat in action and learn from a pro, check out the amazing deep throat porn star, Heather, on her site at ideepthroat.com.

6 **It's a team effort.** While we might separate blow jobs from hand jobs, a finger in the butt from hands on the nuts, the truth is all of these sex acts can work together as a team. Ⓒ Many of the men we surveyed told us that the surest way to bring them off (outside of intercourse) is by mixing all these techniques into one giant climactic bomb. Says Fred, a forty-five-year-old teacher, "I love it when my wife uses one hand to play with my balls, the other stroking my shaft, while her tongue softly whips back and forth on my frenulum. As I get close to orgasm, she squeezes the shaft with increasing pressure and begins to suck the head."

7 **69 is divine.** For mutual satisfaction there is, simply put, nothing better than 69. In this position you are both mouth to genitals, allowing for the simultaneous giving and receiving of oral pleasure. A great advantage of 69 is sometimes you can get so lost in the pleasure you are receiving that you lose your pesky gag reflex and can take him deeper into your mouth than ever.

To get the most from this classic position, experiment with the many variations. Try him on top, you on top, or both of you lying sideways nose to crotch. For a real dirty twist, have your guy lie down with his feet dangling off the edge of the bed, and you climb on top. Ⓓ Then have him sit up, keeping his mouth on your pussy and yours on his cock. Ⓔ You'll now be inverted, so use your hands on the edge

Ⓒ

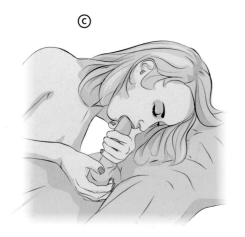

Ⓓ

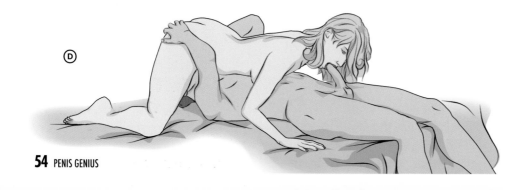

of the bed to support your weight. If he's really strong and you're comfortable with it, wrap your hands around his backside and have him stand up while in position. Ⓕ Either way, the head rush you'll get from being upside down will make your orgasm that much more delightful.

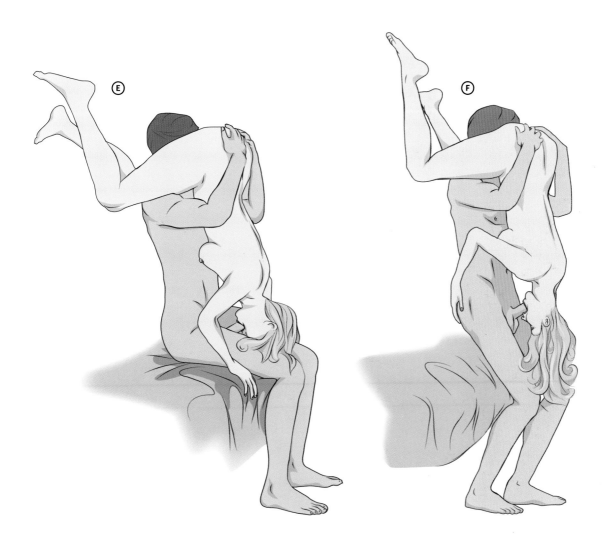

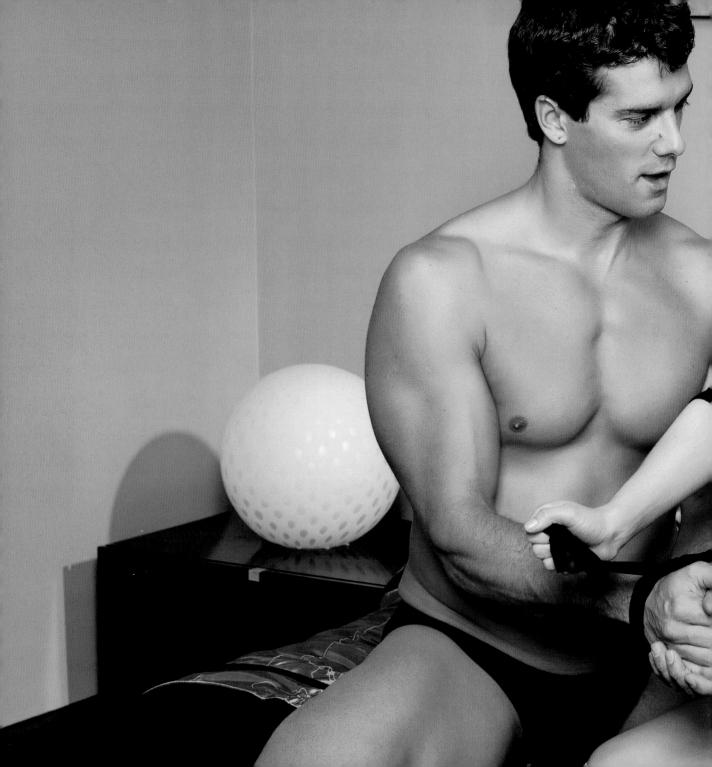

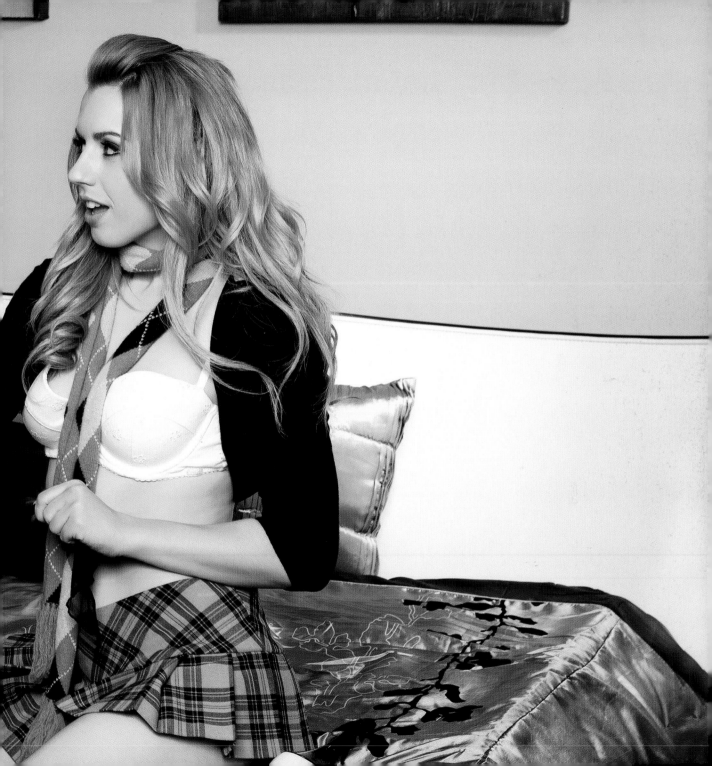

Let's face it: Your guy is an expert at stroking his own shaft. What better way to learn how to handle his hard-on than by asking him to masturbate for you?

GET A HANDLE ON HAND JOBS

Want to wrap him around your finger? Giving a hand job is a simple and fun way to excite your man, make him extra hard, and bring him to a hands-on climax. Just as with the blow job, some girls love giving a hand job and some girls could care less. To all those with friendly fingers out there, we'd like to point out that hand jobs are the go-to move when you want to be discreet (think sexy situations in which you can't remove your own clothing or properly bend over for a nice, sloppy BJ), and they're also perfect for when you want to practice safe sex but don't have a condom.

The Rules

If you can understand and follow these ground rules for jerking him off, he's that much closer to being putty in your hands:

❶ **Take care of your mitts.** Make sure your hands are not overly dry, cracked, or calloused. We don't want to chafe the poor guy!

❷ **The pleasures of lube.** When giving hand jobs, the sky's the limit on which type of lube you can use. Try your favorite sex lube, suntan lotion, sudsy soap in the shower, or whatever you've got on hand. While lube isn't always necessary, it can be lots of fun.

❸ **Let him show you how it's done.** Let's face it: Your guy is an expert at stroking his own shaft. What better way to learn how to handle his hard-on than by asking him to masturbate for you? It's even better than having him try to tell you what he likes. Take, as an example, the hilarious scene from a 2004 Swedish movie called *The Ketchup Effect*, wherein Sebbe (Filip Berg) tries to explain to Sofie (Amanda Renberg) how to give him a hand job. He says, "Imagine you're holding a bottle of ketchup, and you want to get the ketchup out." The response? She takes his penis out of his pants and slaps the end of it like she's trying to slap his sauce out.[35] Ouch! The lesson? Show, don't tell. Follow his lead and match your man stroke for stroke to bring him to a blissful finish.

Tips to Try If You've Mastered the Basic Stroke

For you ladies who've already mastered masturbating your man, here are some genius tips to add to your repertoire:

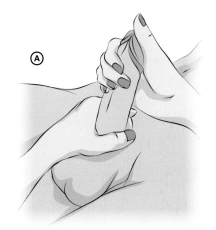

1 **Finger his frenulum and caress his cockhead.** Much like your clit and labia are for you, the frenulum and cockhead (glans) are the most sensitive to touch for him. The frenulum is located on the underside of his shaft; it's that little strip of flesh that connects the top of his shaft to his head. Try gripping his shaft firmly in one hand and pumping up and down, and use your other hand to rub his glans in circles. Ⓐ Gently tease the area with your fingernails, or use your thumb to stroke his frenulum in a short, rhythmic, upward motion from the bottom of the strip to the top.

2 **Use different strokes.** Don't feel like you have to stick to the predictable, basic up-and-down stroke. A little creativity in your touch can be a nice surprise that can bring him to the brink.

3 **Try adding a *twist*:** Instead of stroking in straight lines, wrap your slippery palm around his shaft and twist your wrist left and right as you simultaneously stroke up and down.

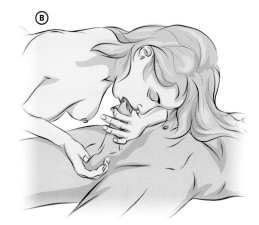

Or try forming a tight *ring* with your thumb and forefinger and push his cockhead through your lubed-up digits. Ⓑ Focus on squeezing his coronal ridge through the tightened space you've made with your fingers while using your other hand to caress his balls.

Tease his shaft with light brushes of your fingertips: Place your palm on his cockhead and let your fingers graze up and down his shaft, just lightly scratching the surface. Your hand will resemble a swimming jellyfish. Ⓒ

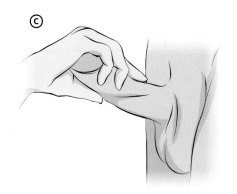

Using a firm grip, wrap your hand around his shaft, beneath the glans, and squeeze and release him in a rhythmic *pulse*. Do *not* stroke your hand up and down. Use your tongue or your other hand to caress his exposed cockhead or massage his testicles while you push him to the edge.

4 **Try some shower fun.** Bring a little thrill to your morning shower by popping in with him while he is warm, wet, and sudsy. For a slippery encounter, use body soap (avoid shampoo) or a few drops of silicone lube. Stand behind him, reach around to take his penis in your hands, and give him a nice rhythmic massage while rubbing your breasts against his back. Keep at it until he spouts, and it will be the perfect start to his workday.

Tips to Try If the Hand Job Just Doesn't Sound Hot

If you think hand jobs sound boring or are too much work, have we got news for you! There are many ways to make slipping his penis between your palms exciting and fun:

1 **Be spontaneous.** Giving a hand job is the perfect sex act for spontaneous fun, as it doesn't require much undressing and can be done quite surreptitiously. If you find yourself in a situation where you don't have any lube (say, in the back row of a nearly empty movie theater), it is still possible to give a knockout hand job. Simply use a featherlight touch. The skin on his penis is much more elastic than you might think, and you can move it without hurting him. Be aware, if you go the lube-free route; make sure you're not stroking him with chapped fingers after a day of rock climbing or gardening without gloves. While lube isn't necessary, your soft skin on his is a must. Says Luke, a sixtysomething writer, "Light, tickling strokes do it for me! No lube needed."

2 **Remember, you don't have to use your hand from beginning to end.** Once you've had fun wrapping your fingers around him, you can always switch to a blow job or intercourse to make him come.

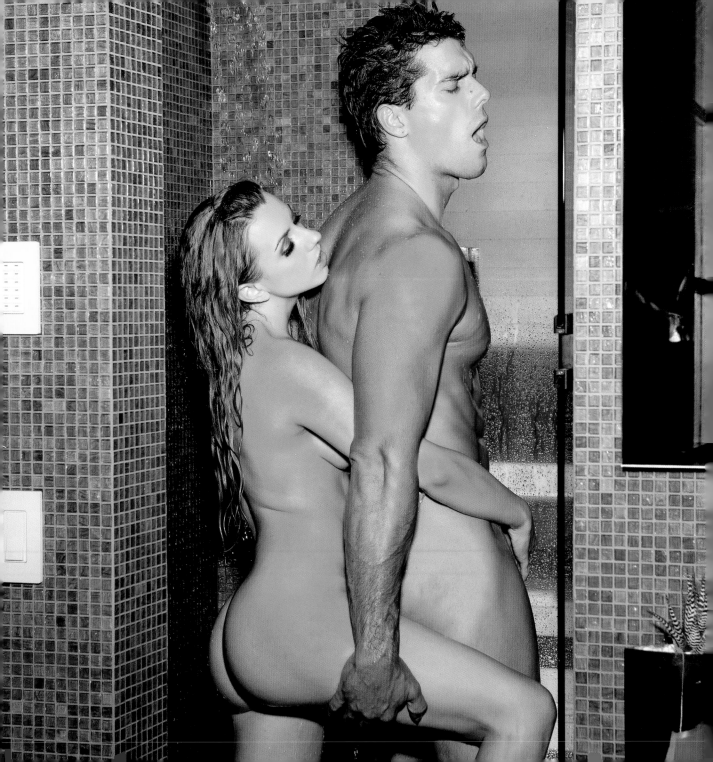

When it comes to sex positions, the majority of men we surveyed prefer Doggy-Style (you on your hands and knees with him penetrating from behind) above all others, followed by Cowgirl (you on top) and Missionary (him on top).

SEXCITING POSITIONS TO BRING TO THE BEDROOM

When it comes to sex positions, the majority of men we surveyed prefer Doggy-Style (you on your hands and knees with him penetrating from behind) above all others, followed by Cowgirl (you on top) and Missionary (him on top). Says Jay, a thirtysomething accountant, "I find that my favorites include Doggy-Style, with my hands gripping and controlling her hips for optimum thrust effectiveness, and good old Missionary. . . . I also enjoy Cowgirl and Reverse Cowgirl (woman on top, facing his feet) with a woman who understands how to move her hips when on top."

Sure, these may be great go-to positions to ensure a satisfying orgasm. But what would happen if you tried something new? We challenge you to try these five fabulous positions that will stimulate his penis in different ways. (For additional positions tailored to the size and shape of your man's package, read chapter six.)

Position #1: Cowboy

If he loves Cowgirl and Missionary, he might just love Cowboy! This position combines the two for penis-pleasing fun. Lie on your back and spread your legs. He straddles your hips on his knees, while keeping his body upright, and penetrates you. Once he's comfortably inside, close your legs for a nice, tight squeeze. This will give you the feeling of fullness, and he'll have the luxury of being able to control the thrusts and spur his way to a powerful climax.

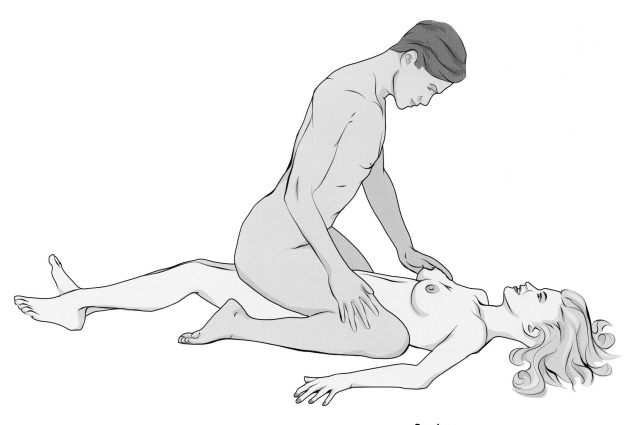

Cowboy

This position allows extra-deep penetration, so don't be surprised if you feel his little head bump up against your back wall. For a little added fun, reach around your thighs and give his testicles a massage as he plunges away.

Position #2: Cuban Plunge

Here's a spicy twist on Missionary: the Cuban Plunge. Start in Missionary and then bring your knees up to your chest, letting your calves rest on his shoulders. This position allows extra-deep penetration, so don't be surprised if you feel his little head bump up against your back wall. For a little added fun, reach around your thighs and give his testicles a massage as he plunges away.

Position #3: Superwoman

Take Doggy-Style up a notch and try Superwoman. Stand and face the edge of the bed (or another sturdy, flat surface, such as your dining room table) and bend over it. Support your torso on the surface and extend your legs in the air behind you so you are positioned like a flying superhero. Your partner enters from between your legs and supports your hips with his arms. Because Superwoman requires a bit of core strength and leg stamina on your part, it can be made easier by doing it in a place where you can push your feet up against a wall. This position is great for his thrusting control, and gives you the delightful feeling of being completely ravished by your man.

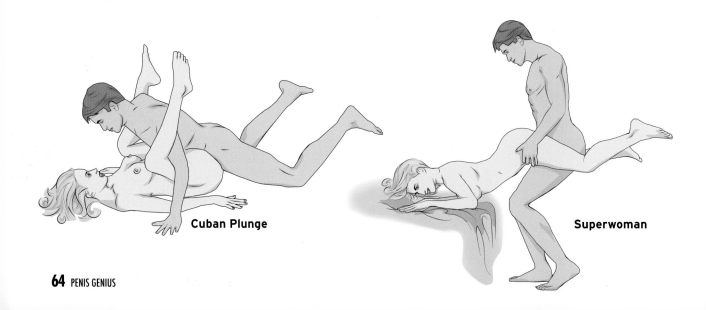

Cuban Plunge

Superwoman

Position #4: Amazon

Let your wild side out to explore the Amazon position. This girl-on-top arrangement will give your man a whole world of new sensations. He lies on his back and draws his knees up to his chest, with his legs slightly spread. You can either squat (if you're strong) or kneel (if your legs tire easily) on either side of his hips and slide onto his cock. Place pillows under your knees if you are too short for this position. The Amazon may make him feel vulnerable, as it completely exposes his nether regions to you, plus he'll have to let you take control because he'll be pinned beneath you. He can caress your tits or tease your clit as you ride him. You can easily reach around to caress his perineum or anus, as well. Also, this is a great position for G-spot stimulation, and because you'll be controlling the thrust and depth of penetration, it's a good go-to move for when you are ready to achieve your orgasm.

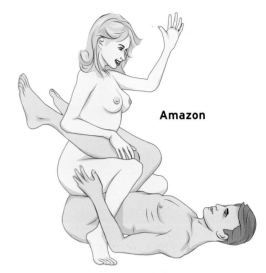

Amazon

Position #5: Bookends

After reading a bit of erotica together, you may want to continue your own sex story by trying Bookends. Kneel facing each other. Spread your legs and have him thrust up into you. If he is much taller than you, he may have to spread his legs wider than yours so he can enter you from below. You can either keep your knees wide for a smooth entry, or squeeze them together to add some friction. Take advantage of being face-to-face by kissing each other and massaging each other's nipples, shoulders, and backs.

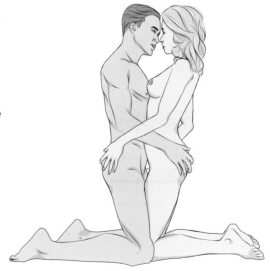

Bookends

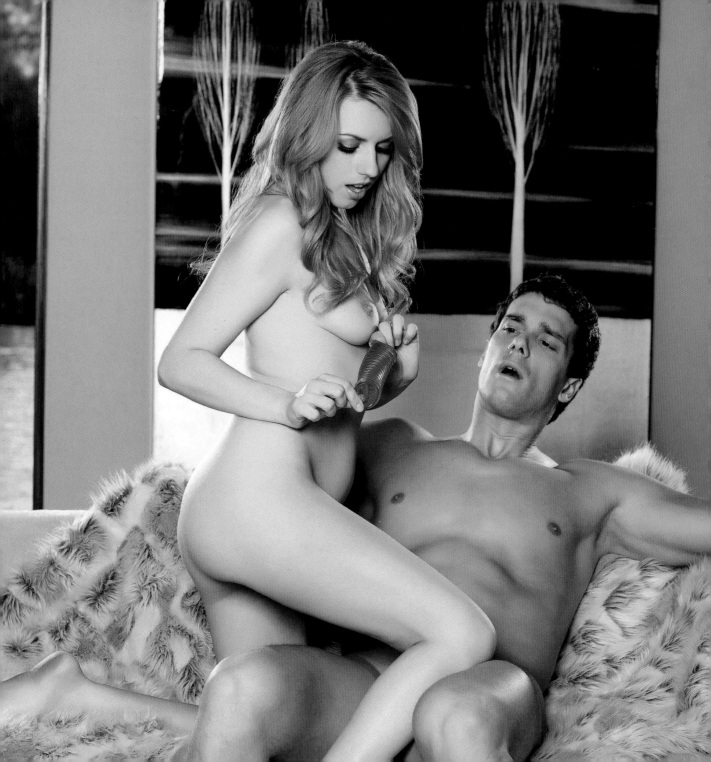

THE JOYS OF SEX TOYS

Masturbation sleeves and cock rings are two categories of sex toys that are made specifically for the penis and can be lots o' fun during playtime. Remember, while he can use these toys during his solo explorations, they're also a great way to add a kinky twist to your partnered sex.

Masturbation Sleeves

Just like your dildo is meant to simulate a penis, masturbation sleeves are designed to simulate a vagina or anus. He uses one by lubing up his penis, slipping the sleeve on, and pumping it up and down his shaft. The devices come in an array of materials, from silicone to ultra-realistic skinlike material. Your guy can choose from sleeve models that range from toylike, colorful tubes to realistic body parts modeled after porn stars. Sleeves are also equipped with different textured interiors, including smooth, ribbed, and wavy, which lend variety to the sensations.

However, be aware that one size does not necessarily fit all, especially if your man is on the larger side of the spectrum. Sophisticated sex toy sites have sizing charts to help you determine which sleeve will best fit your man's equipment. With all the variety out there, it may take you a few tries before you find his perfect match.

Some masturbation sleeves come with their own set of humorous issues, too. Karl, a thirty-four-year-old electrical engineer, says of his toy, "My girlfriend bought me a masturbation sleeve, and it almost feels like the real thing and it's a nice change-up from using my hand. But I don't use it much because my jizz squirts out the opening when I ejaculate, and then I have to go find where it landed." An easy way to solve this messy problem is to have him wear a condom, or you can squeeze the end of the tube closed or put your palm over the top of his head when he comes. Or look for a model that has a closed-off end.

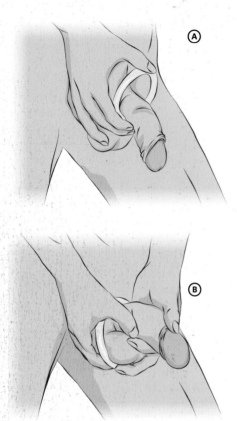

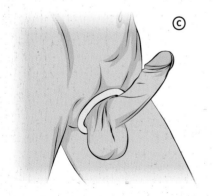

Cock Rings

A cock ring is a delightful device to bring into the bedroom. Traditional cock rings are made of metal or rubber, but newer models come in a multitude of materials with a variety of features and textures. They work by trapping the blood in his penis, which results in larger and longer-lasting erections, so they are particularly handy for guys who worry about the size of their peckers or premature ejaculation.

The key is choosing the right size for your man. The smaller diameter rings trap more blood in his penis, causing more intense erections. But a cock ring novice may freak out when asked to slip his dick into something that looks a lot smaller than his shaft. So when you buy his first cock ring, it's important to choose a ring that is about the same diameter as his erection (a 1.75- to 2-inch [4.4- to 5-centimeter] ring will fit most men). Once he becomes more experienced, he can try something smaller. Don't leave a cock ring on for longer than about twenty minutes at a time, as extended wear can cause nerve damage. Be sure to remove it if he feels any pain or his penis or testicles become cold.

A cock ring should be put on when your man is still flaccid. He should apply a generous amount of lube to his shaft and balls, and then slide the ring all the way to the base of his cock Ⓐ and gently pull his testicles through. ⒷⒸ If he is wary of pulling his testicles through the ring, he can simply wear it at the base of the shaft (although once things get slippery, it may slide off during intercourse). If he's working himself into a metal ring, have him put his testicles in first, one at a time, and then push his flaccid penis through. Another option is to buy a ring that has an opening snap; this way he can just button up after it's on. Be aware that if he gets too excited, there is a chance that the snap will pop open and the ring could fall off during play.

For extra sensation, try using a vibrating cock ring. Just position the vibrating attachment so that it makes contact with your clit.

Sometimes all it takes to add more excitement to your penis handling is adding a little variety to your routine. Trying new positions and techniques, and adding new props to your repertoire, will take you from being a penis layperson to a penis expert.

SCIENTIFICALLY SPEAKING: WHICH LUBE SHOULD YOU USE?

Here's a handy chart to use when picking out the appropriate lube.

	Water-based, no glycerin	Flavored or warming water-based	Silicone-based	Petroleum oil-based
Pros/Cons	Very safe and have multiple uses, but dry out quickly and need to be reapplied frequently	Adds fun sensations, but many flavored/warming lubes contain glycerin, which can cause yeast infections	Is great for water play, is long lasting, but damages certain materials and can stain your sheets	Never dries out, is long lasting, but damages certain materials and can stain your sheets
Vaginal Sex	YES	NO	YES	NO
Oral Sex	YES	YES	NO	NO
Anal Sex	YES	YES	YES	NO
Hand Jobs/ Male Masturbation	YES	YES	YES	YES
Latex Condoms	YES	YES	YES	NO
Silicon Toys	YES	YES	NO	NO
Rubber, Metal, Glass, or Wood Toys	YES	YES	YES	YES

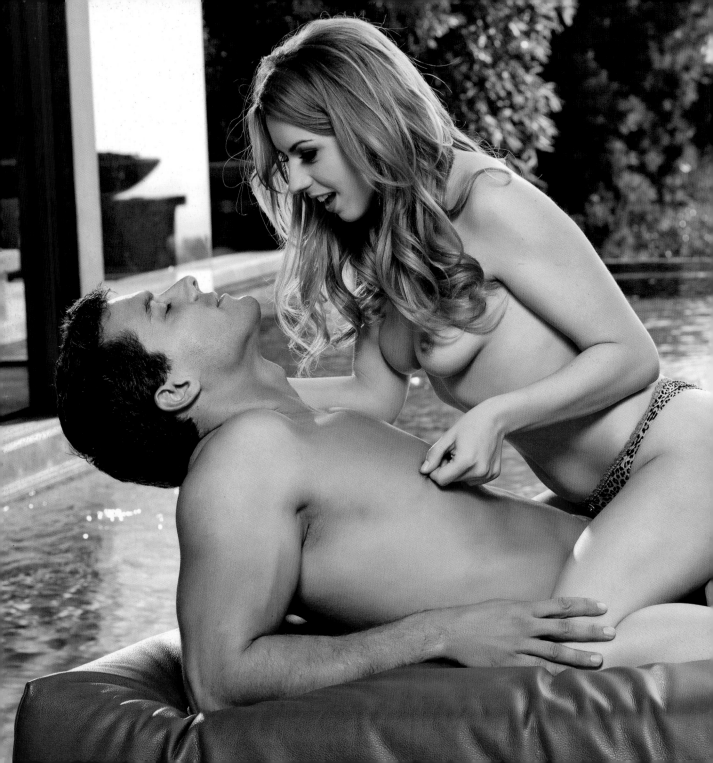

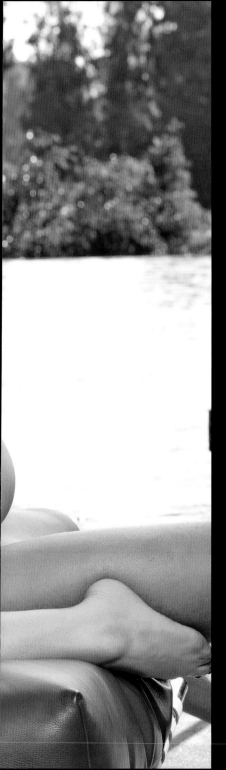

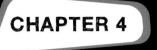

CHAPTER 4

PENIS TEASE: PUSHING HIS OTHER BUTTONS

Ladies, we all know that men are more than just the sum of their penis parts, right? So it makes sense that being a true penis genius means also understanding some of his other buttons, and knowing when and how to push them. These buttons include the nipples, the perineum, the testicles, the prostate, and the anus, and they are all connected to his sexual arousal. Let's talk about how and when to touch these private places in conjunction with your penis play.

LAB WORK: FIND HIS HOT SPOTS

Purpose:
Sure, we know that touching his penis is a big turn on, but where are his other erogenous zones? This lab exercise will help you find the buttons that remotely operate his . . . ahem . . . lever.

What you'll need:
Feather, ice cube, massage oil, red lipstick, blindfold, lab notebook, pencil

The method:

1 Write your lover a note telling him you want to explore his entire body. Include the date and time, and seal it with a lipstick kiss. Put the note in his briefcase or by his toothbrush—somewhere he'll find it later, preferably when you're not with him.

2 When the time for exploration has arrived, obtain permission from your test subject to explore his body. In a sultry whisper, ask him to tell you if there are any spots that are off-limits to your touch. For example, some men are extraordinarily shy when it comes to their butts, while others hate to have their feet touched. It's important that you've got the green light before you explore.

3 Blindfold your subject. This will help him focus his sensate experience on your touch, and will make it feel that much more intense for him.

4 Begin with him in a flaccid (or semi-flaccid) state and do not touch his penis while exploring.

5 Using each of the items (leave lipstick kisses, caress with the feather, trace with the ice cube, and massage with the oil), play with the following areas of his body:
- Back
- Nipples
- Neck
- Earlobes
- Lips
- Feet
- Testicles
- Perineum (that stretch of skin between his testicles and anus)
- Opening of the anus

6 In your lab notebook, record his responses to your touch. Does he cringe? Moan? Laugh? Does he get a hard-on, or does his penis go limp? Does he tell you to stop, or does he beg for more? You might find spots on his body that are more excitable than you ever would have imagined, and you might also find spots to avoid, or to tread lightly upon. Have fun!

7 At the end of the experiment, he should be covered in lipstick kisses from head to toe. If you notice any glaring spots that need attention, take care of those now!

The conclusion:
Through these explorations, you'll discover that his body is covered with erogenous zones. You may have overlooked some of these sensitive spots in your eagerness to get your hands around his hard-on. Add this new knowledge to your sexual library on your way to becoming a penis genius.

But don't let the experimenting end here! Ask him if there are any other tactile sensations he might be curious about. (For example, would he like to donate his body to the study of ticklers or vibrating toys?) The more you experiment, the more you'll be able to truly understand your man's likes and dislikes. Use the information you gather from these experiments to truly master your man's penis pleasure.

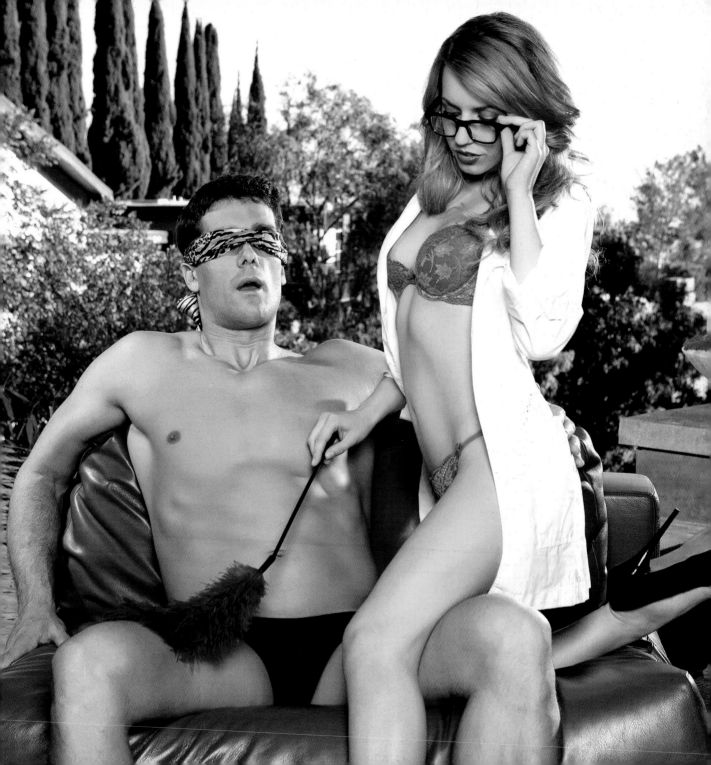

Which parts of your body do you like to have stimulated during intercourse?

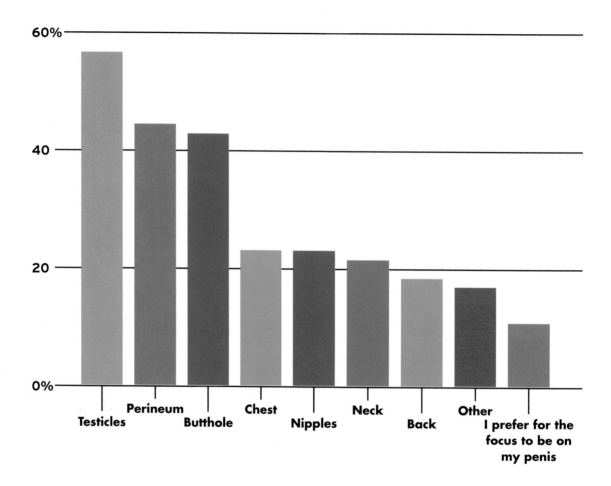

Fifty-six percent of our men say they love having their testicles played with during intercourse. What's in the "Other" category? Abs, prostate, legs, ears, and feet.

TANTALIZE HIS TESTICLES

Testicles reside in the scrotal sack that hangs just below his penis. At first glance, they may look as foreign as those furry monsters from *Fraggle Rock*, but as a major center of male pleasure, it would do you well to become acquainted with these little guys.

In our survey, a whopping 56 percent of men reported that they love having their testicles stimulated, especially in conjunction with intercourse. Says thirty-three-year-old Lenny, "My girlfriend will sometimes reach down between us and lightly cup and run her fingers over my sack and sometimes go as far as my perineum and anus. . . . It feels absolutely amazing."

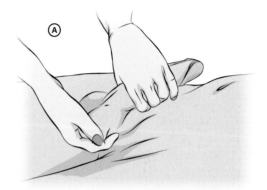

Sexy Techniques to Try

❶ Incorporate the testicles into your blow job technique. Give them a tender squeeze or lube up and massage them very gently in your palm as you tongue his shaft.

❷ Try gently tugging down on the testicles in a milking motion. Some men love the feeling of having the scrotum and balls gently stretched. Be sure to ask him if he likes it. Ⓐ

❸ Use a feather or your fingernails to tickle and tease.

❹ Lap each testicle with your tongue, one at a time, and then oh-so-gently bring one into your mouth with your lips and tongue. Suckle it in your mouth before you release it, and do the same to the other one. Ⓑ (For more ideas, see chapter one.)

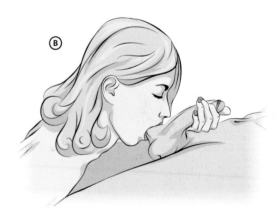

Contraindication Warning

The testicles are extremely sensitive to pain (just as your ovaries would be if they had to hang outside the body). Never poke, knock, or squish them (or it will be a cold shoulder and lights out tonight).

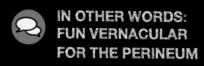
RIDE THE PERINEUM HIGHWAY

The perineum is that little stretch of pleasurable highway that runs from his anus to just behind his ball sack. The subcutaneous tissue is sensitive, smooth, and rife with nerve endings. Because it's located below his cock and balls, it's one spot that is easily overlooked. However, men love to have this erogenous zone licked, fingered, and massaged. Forty-four percent of the men we surveyed say they enjoy having their perineum stimulated during sex.

Sexy Techniques to Try

1 To spice up that hand job, gently cup and lift his testicles with one hand as you stroke his shaft with the other. Flatten your tongue and gently lap the length of his perineum, from the edge of his anus to the base of his scrotum. Repeat. Ⓐ

2 Next time you are riding on top like a naughty cowgirl, reach between his legs and place one or two fingers on this lovely morsel of flesh and stroke in circular motions. When you can tell he's close to the brink, use your knuckle to increase the pressure and massage the spot like you're kneading a sexy piece of guy-dough. Be careful not to press too hard, though—you don't want to hurt him. Ⓑ

3 For a completely out-of-this-world sensation, invest in a small vibrating bullet and roll it against his perineum while giving him head. Start at a low level vibration and if he responds with pleasure, turn it up until you slingshot him to the moon.

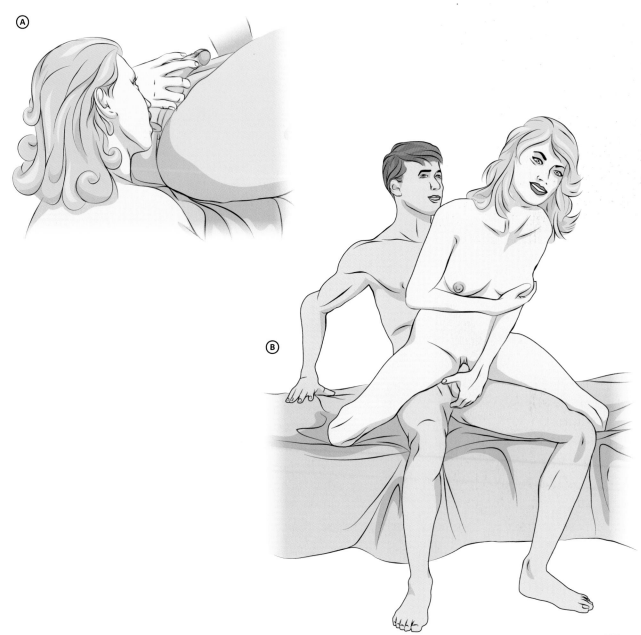

THE BACKDOOR MAN

In our survey, 42 percent of men reported that they enjoy a woman who plays with their butthole. Because this secret space has a large number of nerve endings, the anus is a hugely sensitive erogenous area. Now don't be shy ladies. If your lover loves a little backdoor action, or is even curious about it, just a brush of your finger against the opening can be enough to send some men into la-la land.

Sexy Techniques to Try

1 As you deliver that knockout blow job, gently press the pad of your finger against his anal opening. You can just let your digit rest there, or slowly massage his pucker-hole in circles. Try timing these with the circular swirls of your tongue. Oh la la!

2 If you are a bit more adventurous, take a good dollop of lube and gently explore around the opening before pushing your finger inside. (Be sure you have clipped your nails short and smooth!) Press against the walls of his anus and slowly open the area to your touch. Press your finger in a couple of inches. If you are overcome with the desire to finger-fuck him, make sure you ask him first and go slowly.

3 To kick it up a notch, once he's relaxed to your fingers, slip in a sex toy specifically designed for his butt. Anal beads, butt plugs, and slim dildos designed just for anal penetration are among the toys you might want to stock in your bedside drawer. Be sure that whatever you choose has a wide base or a handle. There is no back wall to the anal canal, and a toy that is not designed for anal pleasure could potentially get lost up there.

4 If you're incredibly adventurous and he's squeaky clean, try pressing your tongue to his bumhole. This is a sure-fire way to take your hand job from ho-hum to holy f$#@!cking cow. (To practice safer sex, use a dental dam during analingus, or even a sheet of plastic wrap.)

5 Don't forget to use a silicone- or water-based lube!

MASSAGE HIS PROSTATE

The prostate can be a source of intense and unique erotic pleasure. When a man ejaculates, the prostate contracts, pulses, and expels the fluid that makes up about a third of his semen. When you massage his prostate by way of his perineum or rectum, you not only stimulate the many nerve endings that surround his prostate, but also encourage and enhance the pleasurable orgasmic contraction. The intensity of his orgasm can be increased two- to threefold with prostate massage.[36]

Follow These Simple Steps for a Perfect Prostate Massage

1. Get his permission! While a lot of men love anal stimulation, some men are anti-backdoor action.

2. Clip your fingernails; nothing is worse than a sharp object up the butt.

3. Have him clean thoroughly. It's not a fun surprise to dip your finger in a hiney full of poo. (Note that this unlikely surprise will only occur if he hasn't thouroughly cleaned after evacuating. The anal canal is only a passageway for his number two; it's not a storage facility.)

4. Slick him up with water- or silicone-based lube.

5. Loosen him up and get him excited by kissing him, playing with his penis, and massaging his perineum and anal opening.

6. Once he's relaxed, slowly push your finger into his tush up to your first knuckle. The pad of your finger should be facing the front side of his body. (A)

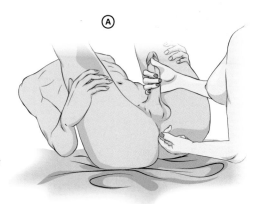

(A)

7. Feel around for hard tissue, about the size of a walnut. Eureka! That's his prostate. When you find it, begin to stroke it by making a "come hither" type of gesture.

8. Continue to play with his cock, kiss him, and encourage him to enjoy himself. You'll know that you've hit jackpot when he starts to pulse around your finger—the beginning contractions of his ejaculation.

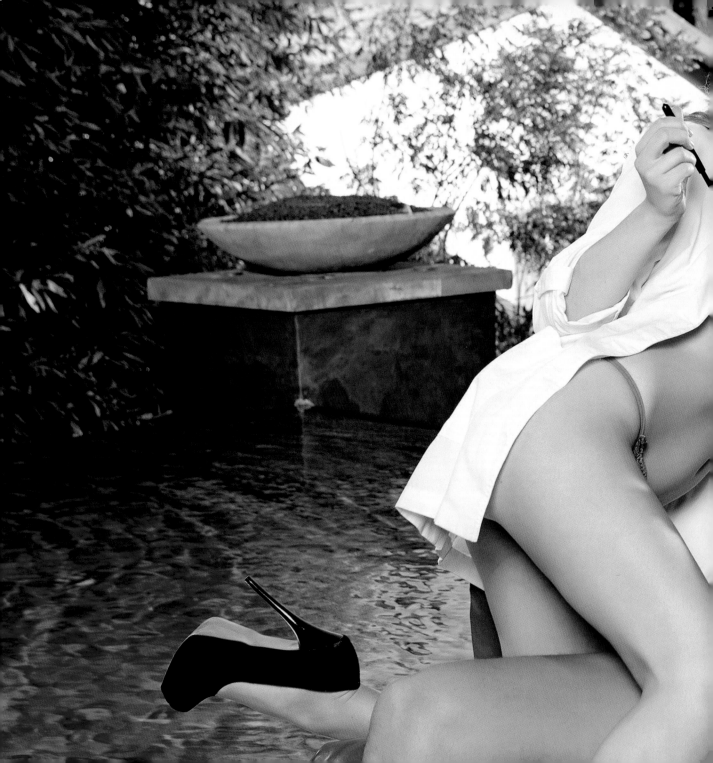

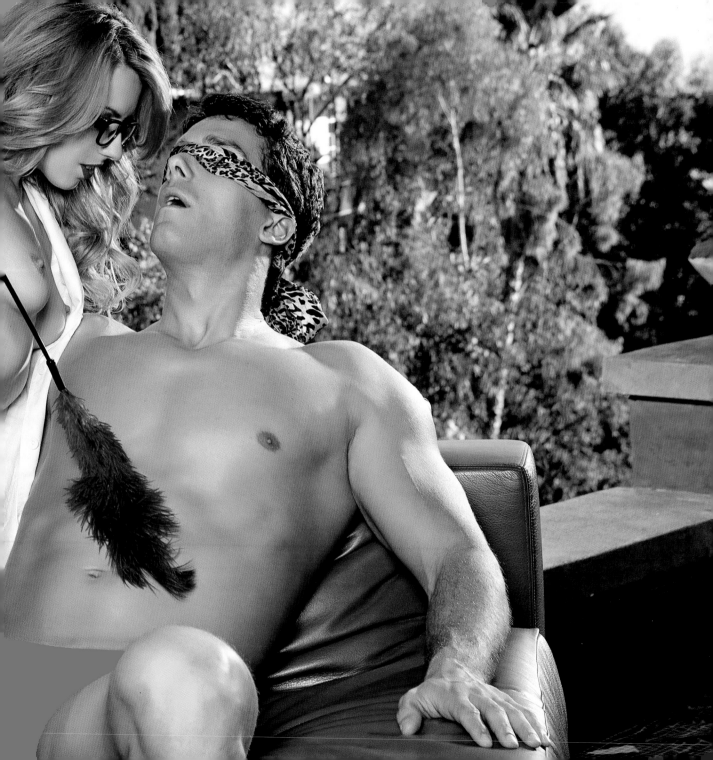

9 If you are uncomfortable putting your finger up his butt, there are a variety of fun prostate massage toys available to purchase. Some you can even put in place and they'll do the "dirty" work while you attend to your preferred body parts.

TITILLATE HIS NIPPLES

In our survey, 61 percent of men reported that their nipples are a particularly sensitive erogenous zone, and 23 percent enjoy nipple stimulation during sex. Says fiftysomething Mark, a civil servant, "While I am inside her, I like her to bite my nipples." Touch his nipples in the same way you enjoy having yours touched.

Sexy Techniques to Try

1 Pinch the nub gently between your thumb and forefinger, and then rotate your fingers clockwise and counterclockwise; ask him if he wants more or less pressure.

2 Roll the nipple under the palm of your hand.

3 Pinch his nipples lightly (or firmly) between your fingers and tug on them, or even bite them.

4 Lick and suck those babies to erection.

5 Rest your hands on his chest and, using just your thumbs, rub his nipples in an upward stroke from bottom to top.

6 If you are both feeling particularly adventurous, try using one of the various nipple-teasing toys available at sex toy stores. Many of them come with suctioning, vibrating, or pinching action. Just secure one of these little suckers onto his nips, and your hands and mouth will be free to go to town on the rest of his body.

EROTIC MASSAGE: A ROLE-PLAYING GAME

An erotic massage can be just what the doctor ordered. Add a little role-playing to this activity to make it a truly sexy experience.

Here is how the story might go: Pretend you are a professional massage therapist, and your lover is a new customer. Set up a massage area on your bed; be sure to cover it with a towel or a set of sheets that you don't mind spilling a little oil on. Set up the room with dim lights and inviting music. Instruct your "customer" to fully undress and lie facedown beneath the sheet, and then leave the room. When he is situated, politely knock on the door and return to the room.

Start by folding the sheet down to expose his back, leaving his buttocks covered. Gently stroke his back with your fingertips. Ask him where he is holding tension. Get to know him a little—ask him what he does for a living and whether he is in a relationship. Tell him he has a sexy back. Ask him if he lifts weights. Pour a tablespoon of massage oil onto your hands and rub them together to warm it up. Slather it onto his skin. Ask him how it feels. Start to massage it in, rubbing up and down his spine and in circles around his back and shoulders. Ask him if it's okay to rub his butt, and then slowly pull the sheet down to expose it. Add more oil and begin to rub his behind, kneading it with your knuckles and squeezing it in your fingers. Part his legs and occasionally, "accidentally," brush your fingers against his scrotum and crack. Ask him if he would like to turn over so that you can take care of his front side. When he turns over, massage his chest and abs, but don't touch his penis. Not until he asks you to!

It's a great pleasure to discover all those little off-the-penis parts that give your man a thrill in the sack. Enjoy, be safe, and have fun!

SCIENTIFICALLY SPEAKING: WHY DO MEN HAVE NIPPLES?

Plainly put, nipples are like hands, knees, or eyebrows. Everyone has them because they are not a sex-specific characteristic (as vaginas and penises, testicles and ovaries are). When he was but a three-week-old embryo, your man's nipples developed, a full four weeks before any of his male sex characteristics did. Men's nipples come complete with milk ducts, just like yours. And given enough estrogen, he potentially could lactate.[38]

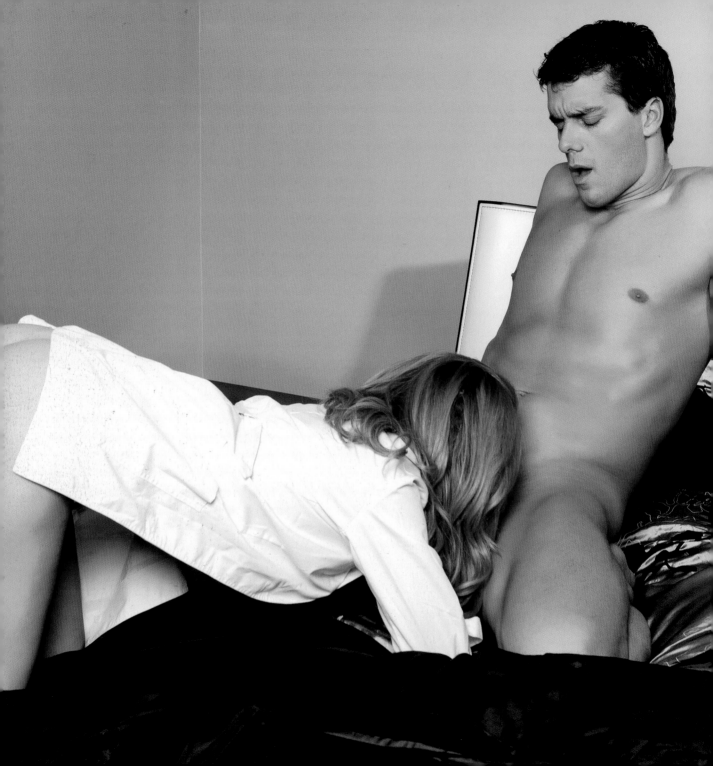

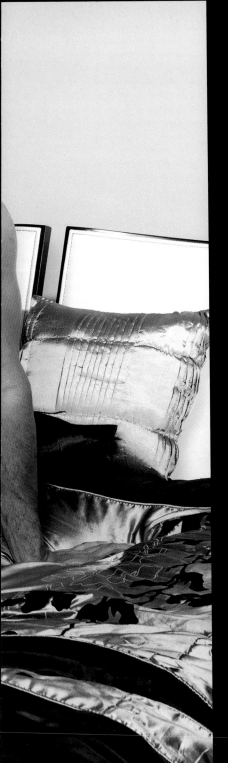

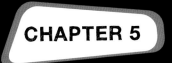
CHAPTER 5

CIRCUMCISED VS. UNCIRCUMCISED: WHAT MODEL DOES YOUR MAN HAVE?

Your man's penis will look, and sometimes react, differently to stimulis based on whether he is circumcised. Do you know what model penis your man has? You might want to take a second look.

Kerri, a thirty-three-year-old electrician, tells us, "My boyfriend and I have been intimate for about three months. It wasn't until recently when I saw his flaccid penis for the first time that I realized that I was dating an uncircumcised man. I've been 'down there' so many times during sex and never noticed his foreskin! It shocked me, but I was pleasantly surprised because I'd heard so many rumors that sex with uncircumcised men was gross. He's actually the best I've ever had. Whether or not it has to do with his intact penis, I'm not sure."

Let's look closely and observe the difference between an uncircumcised cock (**MODEL A**) and a circumcised cock (**MODEL B**).

In model A, you'll see when flaccid, the foreskin of the uncircumcised penis completely covers the glans. The urethra of the penis may peek out the end and wink at you, or the foreskin may extend beyond the urethra and look like a deflated balloon.

As his penis hardens under the effects of your genius, you'll notice that the foreskin pulls back and settles under his head, resembling a tube sock. When fully erect, the inner foreskin remains beneath the glans, and the outer layer of the foreskin stretches to the middle of his shaft. Visually, a fully erect, uncut penis looks similar to a cut penis, because the glans is fully visible and the foreskin is taut around the shaft.[39]

In model B, you'll see that a flaccid circumcised penis looks more like a mushroom, with its exposed, helmetlike head. When fully erect, the entire penis fills with blood and expands, making the glans look fuller and the shaft look taut.

Which model is more appealing? It's a simple matter of personal aesthetics. Says Renee, a forty-eight-year-old teacher, "I prefer a circumcised cock; it looks better to me. An uncircumcised penis just looks like a bald guy with a turtleneck pulled up over his face . . ." Contrarily, twentysomething Joanne says, "I generally prefer the look, feel, and smell of the uncircumcised penis."

WHICH PENIS FEELS MORE PLEASURE?

The argument about which penis feels more pleasure (cut or uncut) continues to be waged in both science and popular culture. Circumcised men argue that having a more exposed glans allows it to be more easily stimulated. Uncircumcised men say that because their glans is protected from daily chafing, when it does come out to play, it's extra sensitive to touch. However, men who've opted to be circumcised later in life have reported a decrease in sensitivity, and these men may be the ones who can give us the best insight into the matter.

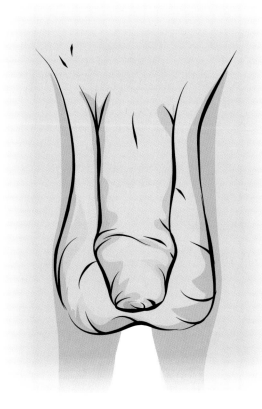

MODEL A

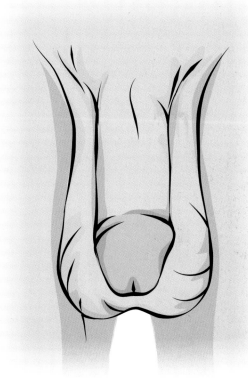

MODEL B

SCIENTIFICALLY SPEAKING: WHAT IS THE PURPOSE OF THE FORESKIN?

One of the better analogies we've come across is to think of the foreskin like an eyelid. Just as an eyelid covers, cleans, and protects the eyeball, the foreskin, when intact, does the same for the glans. In addition, like the inside of the eyelid, the underside of the foreskin is lined with a mucous membrane that secretes emollients, lubricants, and protective antibodies (which makes for extra-slippery, wet sex). The foreskin also contains approximately 240 feet (73 meters) of nerve fibers and tens of thousands of specialized nerve endings (which is one reason some believe sex feels better to an uncut man).

In the 1960s, there was a common belief that circumcised men have better control over their ejaculations (perhaps due to less sensitivity). A study by Masters and Johnson compared thirty-five circumcised men with thirty-five uncircumcised men in an attempt to disprove the theory. They found "no clinically significant difference could be established between the circumcised and the uncircumcised glans." Further, they noted that when aroused, the glans is often fully exposed to touch, so the foreskin does little to protect it from stimulation during sex.[42] The lesson here? It's really anybody's guess as to who feels more pleasure. What we do know from experience is that most men love sex, no matter what model penis they're working with.

If you've had experience with both circumcised and uncircumcised men, did you notice any difference in the following:

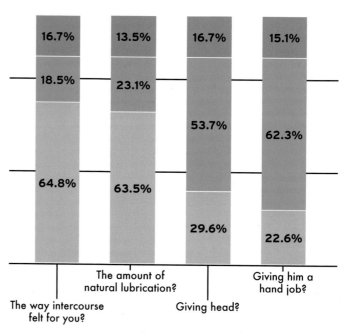

Women found little difference between uncircumcised and circumcised men when having intercourse, but noticed a big difference when giving hand jobs and blow jobs.

WHAT DOES CIRCUMCISION MEAN FOR YOUR SEX LIFE?

What are the differences between playing with a cut versus an uncut cock? While some women can hardly distinguish between the two, others are attuned to the different pleasures each has to offer. Here are some of the discrepancies you might notice (that is, if you're paying close attention!).

Circumcision and Hand Jobs

In our survey, 62.3 percent of women reported a noticeable difference when giving hand jobs to uncircumcised verses circumcised cocks. With an intact foreskin, there is little need for lubrication when giving a hand job thanks to the natural lubrication generated by the mucous membranes in the foreskin. Tina, a twenty-eight-year-old restaurant reviewer says, "It's easier to give a hand job to an uncircumcised man because I can grip the foreskin and slide it."

Says Natasha, a thirty-seven-year-old writer, "Hand jobs are easier to give [when a man is uncircumcised] due to the foreskin. This has been made obvious to me because my current partner was circumcised during our relationship so I have had the experience of both before and after."

With a circumcised penis, you'll want to lube up your palm so that the shaft slides against the skin of your hand, or you can use a featherlight touch. Ⓐ With an uncircumcised penis, the foreskin generates its own lube and glides easily along the shaft as if it were a natural masturbation sleeve; all you have to do is slide it up and down. (For more information on giving great hand jobs, see chapter three.)

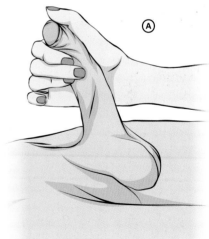

Ⓐ

Circumcision and Giving Head

The biggest complaint women report when it comes to giving head is that sometimes a man doesn't keep his junk nice and clean. Cleanliness is sexiness. This is true whether a man is circumcised or not; after all, your tongue and nose are so involved in the oral experience, a tasty and yummy smelling gent is always preferable.

Uncircumcised men naturally generate a pungent substance called smegma (women produce the same secretion around their labia and clit). Smegma is made from shed skin cells and body secretions and acts as a natural lubricant. When it first develops, it's often clear or whitish and moist and smooth, but if it's allowed to build up, it becomes more of a chunky, cheesy substance.[44] If your lover is uncut, he should bathe and wash regularly and know how to pull the foreskin back to clean out the area. (Parents beware, the foreskin should *not* be retracted before puberty, so this is not meant to be part of a child's bathing ritual, as it can cause urinary tract infections.)

Let's assume you dive into his drawers and he's sporting a squeaky clean woody. What's the difference between **MODEL A** and **MODEL B (see page 87)** as far as oral sex is concerned? More than half (53.7 percent) of women we surveyed say they can tell a big difference when giving head to an uncircumcised man. Libby, a twenty-four-year-old aesthetician raves, "I could entertain myself for hours with a foreskin; it's like unwrapping a present over and over again . . . and you can work pure magic orally." This magic comes from the unique sensations you can bring to your uncut man. The opening of the foreskin is particularly sensitive, and a good tease with your tongue into the entrance can cause bedroom earthquakes. Ⓑ Some men like it when you pull the foreskin all the way down before giving oral (this gives you full access to his glans and frenulum), while other men find their glans to be supersensitive, so they prefer you to suck on the foreskin or just be extra-gentle with the head.

Other women are smitten with model B. Says Lori, a thirtysomething upholsterer, "When giving head, I have found that the head of the circumcised penis is slightly less sensitive than an uncircumcised penis. I personally prefer circumcised penises because they offer a more tactile experience when giving head, as there is never any excess skin." The sensitive frenulum and coronal ridge are fully exposed on circumcised men, and they just beg for you to lick and love them as part of your oral play. (For more information on giving great head, read chapter three.)

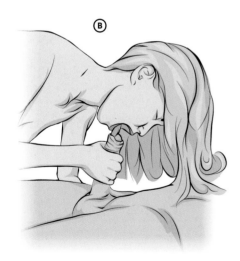

Ⓑ

Circumcision and Intercourse

In our survey, 65 percent of women say they feel no difference between cut and uncut cock during intercourse. Perhaps this is because our vaginas aren't as discriminating as our fingertips and tongues. However, 18.5 percent say there is something to it. Word on the street indicates that the uncircumcised man's penis is a bit more sensitive than his circumcised counterpart, especially around his glans. Women report that the extra sensitivity leads model A men to use slower, gentler strokes. Says Gina, a fortysomething journalist, "Uncircumcised men (which I prefer) have very sensitive heads, and they're very soft, too. Intercourse with uncircumcised men seems to be a lot more sensual. Maybe because the uncircumcised man gets more sensation with each thrust?" Twentysomething Mandy says, "The overall sensation of the sex act feels moister and less abrasive."

However, other women prefer the action they receive from their model B lovers. Says Trish, a forty-three-year-old accounting executive, "Being English, I've been with uncircumcised men for most of my life. When I met my current (American) partner, I was delighted with the absolute rough sex he gives me. He seems to need more friction, and uses rapid strokes that drive me absolutely bananas."

Just like size, shape, angle, and function, the foreskin or lack thereof is yet another characteristic that makes your man's cock unique. Whatever you find behind your man's zipper, you should learn about, experiment with, and enjoy his unique pleasure potential.

LAB WORK: COMPARE AND CONTRAST

Purpose:

Who feels more pleasure? A debate wages about whether circumcised or uncircumcised men feel more sensation during sex. Because sex is such a subjective experience, and most men enjoy it regardless of their condition, it may be impossible for us to put an end to this debate (at least in this book). However, courageous, budding penis geniuses everywhere can take matters into their own hands. Do your own lab work at home, and then get together with as many female lab partners as possible to compare notes to see if your cut partner reacts differently than your girlfriends' uncut partners (or vice versa). In fact, the more men you compare, the better. If you're single and have access to both an uncut and a cut partner, you have even greater opportunity to collect data. Of course, if you do opt to compare multiple partners, be sure to practice the safest sex possible.

What you'll need:

A timer, one or more circumcised men, one or more uncircumcised men, condoms and/or a few willing co-scientist girlfriends, lab notebook, pencil, white lab coat, and a bottle of wine

The method:

1 For the best results from this experiment, you'll need to tap into whatever strict persona you think your lover will find sexiest: Each sex act must be executed as close to identically as possible for each man, so you'll need to inspire your man to follow the guidelines of the experiment. Whether it's that naughty-but-demanding school teacher he's always fantasized about, or a masked dominatrix dressed in black leather, play the part to make sure he follows the rules.

2 Each step of the experiment should be executed in the dark, in the bedroom, and in the same position every time. Inform your man of the rules and let him know you will be timing each sex act that you perform together. Keep it straightforward. If he behaves and does as you ask, tell him you'll reward him later. All lab partners must do the same.

3 Time your blow jobs. On average, how long does each man take to ejaculate? Does the uncut partner come sooner than the cut partner? Or is it the reverse?

4 Skip the foreplay (on him at least) and time your intercourse. Is either partner an eight-minute man? Does one last longer than the other?

5 Using the experiment devised in chapter one, compare which spots are more sensitive on which partner. For example, you may find that your circumcised partner is more sensitive on the head, while your girlfriend's uncircumcised partner has a highly reactive foreskin.

6 In one scientific study, researchers found that uncircumcised men had less sensitive forearms than their circumcised counterparts.[45] Why this may be so, we're unsure. But it could be a fun test to try. Try pinching the forearms of your lovers to see who gives you the bigger reaction.

7 Also observe which experience is more pleasurable for you and why. Which penis do you find to be a smoother ride? Do you orgasm reliably with either one?

8 Try doing each of the above steps on multiple occasions, writing down extensive notes each time.

The conclusion:

Organize a girls' night, bring lab notebooks, and pop open the bottle of wine! Compare and contrast your findings. You may note similar results and finally have an answer for the great debate, but even if you don't, talking sex with girlfriends is always great fun.

WHERE DID CIRCUMCISION ORIGINATE?

Circumcision has been in practice for thousands of years. Egyptians left evidence as early as 2300 BC that they performed male genital alteration rituals as a rite of passage at the onset of puberty. Jews continue the practice of circumcision as a religious covenant that harks back to biblical days. Muslim tradition also honors circumcision, as the prophet Mohammed (who, according to some legends, was born without a foreskin) taught that circumcision is customary for men, and fathers should have their sons look as they are.[46] Interestingly, a popular reason that many nonreligious fathers opt to circumcise their sons is so that their babies will look as they do.

In the late nineteenth century United States, circumcision arose as a fight against "masturbatory insanity." It finds its roots in a publication written by Dr. John Harvey Kellogg (of Corn Flakes fame), titled *Treatment for Self-Abuse and its Effects* (1888). He writes, "A remedy for masturbation which is almost always successful in small boys is circumcision. The operation should be performed by a surgeon without administering an anesthetic, as the brief pain attending the operation will have a salutary effect upon the mind, especially if it be connected with the idea of punishment."[47] Although most of us in present day haven't read this questionable work, somehow circumcision has maintained its popularity in the United States, while most other Western countries have all but abandoned the practice.

If your man was born in the United States, he is likely to be circumcised, as the procedure has been routinely performed in hospitals since about 1930. Circumcision peaked in 1975 when about 93 percent of newborn boys were cut; today that number is down to about 80 percent, which is still a far higher percentage than in Europe where only about 1 percent of newborns are circumcised.[48] Indeed, 76 percent of the men we surveyed reported they are circumcised. Today circumcision is becoming less popular as questions about its benefits have emerged.

Also, because American Academy of Pediatrics guidelines now say that circumcision is unnecessary, some health insurers are calling it a "cosmetic procedure," which means they may not cover the cost.[49]

Circumcision is generally considered to be a safe procedure, with reports of less than 1 percent of cases being "botched" jobs. However, as with any body modification surgery, complications can arise, such as hemorrhaging, infections, and scarring.[50]

On very rare occasions, circumcision surgery can go very, very wrong. One famous example occurred in 1966 when a boy named Bruce Reimer lost his penis to circumcision by the uncommon cauterization method. His parents decided he couldn't live a healthy life as a male and decided to reassign his gender with the aid of psychologist Dr. John Money of Johns Hopkins University. Money, who was working on gender identity studies at the time, took the boy on as a case study to support his theory of gender neutrality and called it the "John/Joan case." Bruce's testicles were surgically removed, and he was renamed Brenda and raised as a girl. Later in life Brenda redefined himself as a man named David, but became so depressed due to financial and marital troubles that he eventually committed suicide in 2004. With horror stories like this one to support the case, some people argue strenuously against circumcision, and go so far as to call it genital mutilation akin to the removal of a girl's clitoris (a surgery that is still performed in parts of Africa).

Ultimately, parents still have the choice when they have a son as to whether to circumcise him. Fifty-two percent of the men in our survey say that they will circumcise their sons (or already have done so). It's important to do your research and make the best decision for you and your family based on medical information as well as your specific religious or cultural considerations.

 FAMOUS PENIS: JOHN WAYNE BOBBITT

Who can forget the grotesque tale of John Wayne Bobbitt and his severed penis? In 1993, citing marital abuse, Lorena Bobbitt severed her husband's penis with a kitchen knife while he slept. She disposed of it in a far-off field, but after realizing what she had done, she helped authorities find the missing unit. Doctors reattached it to John during a six-hour surgery. John went on to capitalize on his ordeal by starring in "John Wayne Bobbitt Uncut," a poorly acted porn film (directed by famous huge-dick porn star Ron Jeremy) that reenacted how he got his "severance package" and, with the assistance of sexy pornographic nurses, went on to prove to the world that "it still works."

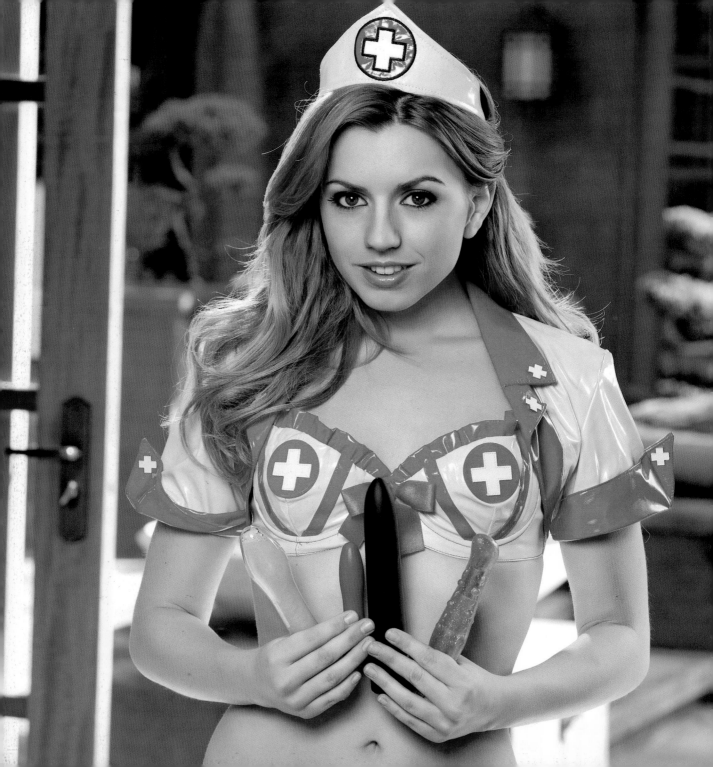

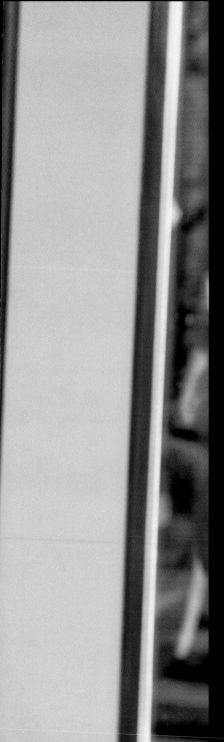

CHAPTER 6

ON SHAPES AND SIZES: PERFECT POSITIONS FOR ALL PENIS PROPORTIONS

Just like fingerprints, no two penises are exactly alike, but most fit into certain broad categories of physical attributes. You may find yourself with a long, slender drink of water, or you may snag yourself a short but rotund specimen. We'll tell you about the best sexual positions you can try to maximize or minimize penetration for the different sizes and shapes of dicks you may come across.

LAB WORK: MEASURING UP

Purpose:

To determine what type of tool he's got beneath his belt. Is it the Hulk or a Maverick? Or something else entirely? This lab exercise provides a playful way to get to know your guy's little guy a little better.

What you'll need:

A ruler, piece of string, lab notebook, pencil, white lab coat (lingerie optional), sexy spectacles, red lipstick, surgical gloves, and high heels

The method:

❶ It's time to play doctor! Put on your sexy white lab coat, some pretend (or real) spectacles, red lipstick, and high heels. Don't forget to snap on your surgical gloves. Have your patient step into your office. First, measure his flaccid penis. Have your guy stand at the edge of a table or counter and rest his cock on the surface. Do not stretch his penis out; just let it rest comfortably, yet as straight as possible. Place the ruler alongside his penis. Write down your measurements.

❷ Flash your naked booty or sexy lingerie from beneath your lab coat, eliciting his arousal. Use your mouth or hands as necessary to facilitate full erection. Once engorged, measure the full length of the *underside* of his cock by placing the ruler at the base of his penis where the testicles connect to the shaft. Write down your measurements.

❸ Finally, take the piece of string and wrap it around his shaft about midway between his glans and testicles to determine the circumference (or girth) of your lover's erection. Don't squeeze too tightly. Pinch the endpoint of the string, and then extend it and measure the length with your ruler. Write down your measurements.

❹ Note the angle of his dangle. Does he curve right? Left? Up? Down? Does his angle change when he is flaccid versus when he is erect? Write down your observations.

❺ Lavish him with praise and adoration. Men are very sensitive when it comes to penis size. Make him feel good about himself by commenting on his perfect penis. In our survey of 285 men, 40 percent reported sporting a 6-inch (15.2-centimeter) penis. Scientists say that the American average length is between 5.25 and 5.5 inches (13.3 and 14 centimeters). But don't let him get hung up on the numbers. This exercise isn't really about comparing him to other guys; it's about deciding how to best play with his member.

The conclusion:

Using your lover's measurements, determine into which of the following categories your guy's penis best fits and read on to try out the sex positions prescribed, based on his specific anatomy.

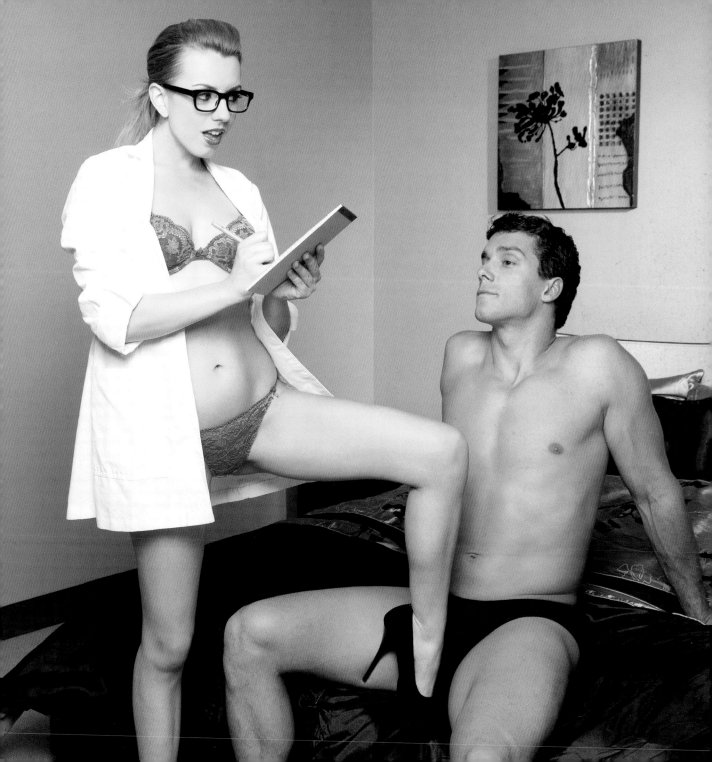

SCIENTIFICALLY SPEAKING: WHAT IS PHALLOPHILIA?

Phallophilia is a psychological term that describes a person's (sometimes unhealthy) obsession with large penises. In pop culture, these people are referred to as size queens, a name that was coined in the gay community but has expanded to include anyone—straight, gay, or otherwise—who prefers oversized dicks. Size queens often refuse to partner with men of smaller proportions, which may have the unfortunate consequence of limiting their relationship opportunities to rude dudes with monster cocks.

From our conversations with women, we know that each one has her own definition of penis perfection. Some love nothing more than a giant cock, others like a more moderate member, or one with a definite left-hand bend, and still others love whatever comes attached to their sweetheart. It's all a question of how well the two puzzle pieces (yours and his) fit together to maximize mutual pleasure. Says forty-six-year-old K.B., "The best penis for me—in any position—is always the one that's about an inch shorter than my pussy and several inches wider. When we get it all slick and I'm all wet, it feels good to still have to force it a bit to get it in. I have to admit that I hate too-long penises for ANY position. My uterus is happy in her present location. No sense in making the old girl relocate!"

Note that the following penis sizes and suggested positions are generalized examples to try with your partner. It is only through your own exploration that you and your partner(s) will find what works best for your unique anatomies.

THE HULK

(At least 8 inches [20.3 centimeters] in length and 5 inches [12.7 centimeters] in circumference)

Unzipping a man's trousers to discover the Hulk lurking in his boxers (minus the green skin and bad attitude) can be an exciting or an alarming experience, depending on who you are. For some women, there's just nothing as delightful as being filled to capacity (and then some), while other women may find the Hulk intimidating, overwhelming, or just downright painful.

Perfect Positions

If you find that your guy is too large for your dainty parts, try riding him in any variation of the girl-on-top positions, which will allow you to control the depth of his penetration. **Cowgirl**[53] is the most basic of these positions: Your man lies down on a flat surface and you straddle his penis, facing him and keeping your knees on either side of his hips. For a variation, ride him **Reverse Cowgirl**. This position is similar to Cowgirl, but you mount him facing backward so that you are looking at his feet. In this position, he gets a titillating view of your behind. If you require even less of his penis inside while riding, try the **Pearly Gates (see pages 102-103):** Start in Reverse Cowgirl and then lie back so you are resting against his chest. This will help limit his penetrative range.

Another great option for coupling with a guy who is extremely well-endowed is **Teaspoons.** Ⓐ In this position, you stand on your knees with your legs spread wide. Your guy kneels behind you and penetrates you from behind. This position not only limits his depth and allows you to spread wide enough to accept his girth, but it also gives him the control over thrusting that he won't get with the girl-on-top positions. For a supersexy twist, he can reach around you to rub your clit and play with your breasts.

However, be careful here *not* to bend over into Doggy Style, which is where you lean forward and put your hands on the floor, as that position provides for incredibly deep penetration and he will be more likely to hit your cervix and the back of your uterus. Ouch!

Tasty Tips

For your pleasure, you should be excited and lubricated no matter what size your guy is, but when partnering with the Hulk, it's even more important to be fully aroused. Enjoying a warm-up orgasm via toy play or oral sex prior to penetration can help "loosen" you up and prepare you to accommodate his full size. Amanda, thirty-two, says, "I'm petite and can barely take an average-sized cock. I was recently with a well-endowed man. As long as my mind was on it, he would not fit. He went down on me until I came, held me still enough while I thrashed around, out of my mind, and slipped into me. Well, slipped isn't the right word . . . but before I knew it, there he was."

You can also try slowly stretching yourself during foreplay by using a sequence of toys that range from your ideal size to something close to his size before attempting to accommodate the Hulk. Or ask him to use his fingers to massage and stretch you open beforehand, starting with one digit and graduating up to four fingers. What fun!

Ⓐ **Teaspoons**

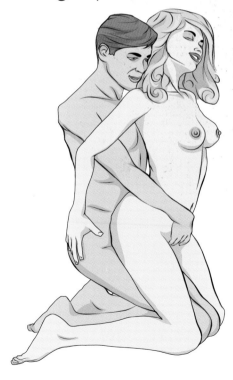

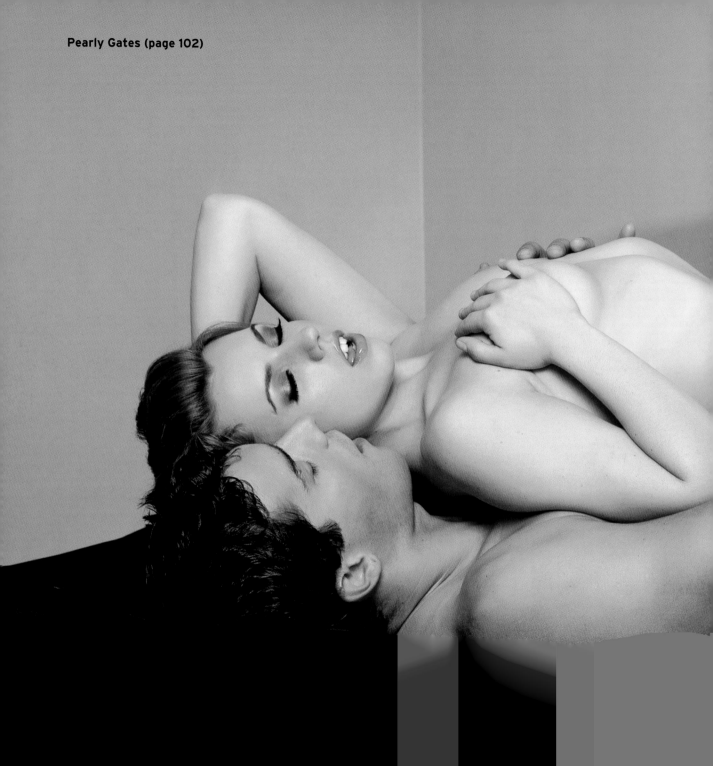

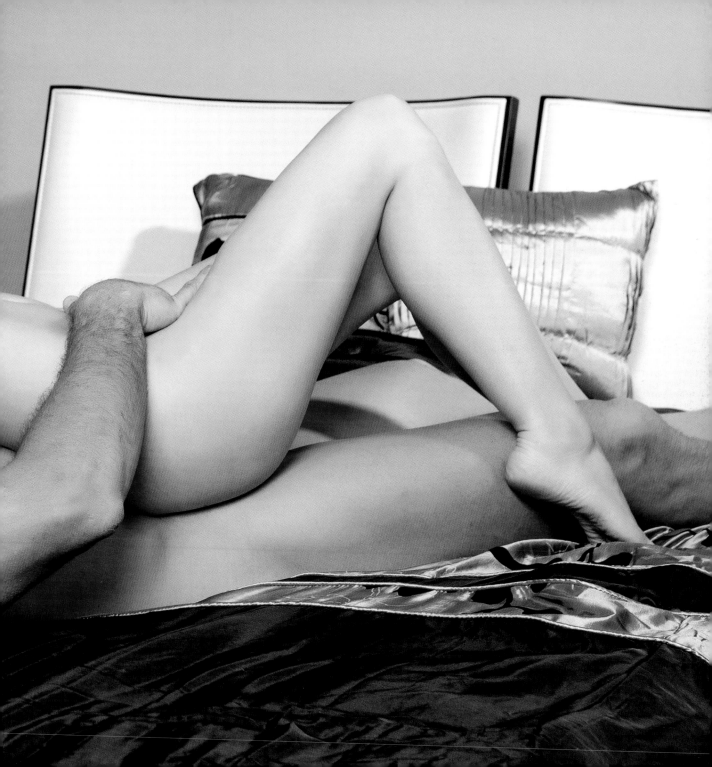

In a survey conducted by the Department of Obstetrics and Gynecology at the Groningen University Medical Center in the Netherlands, researchers asked a group of women who had recently given birth to discuss theiår preferences on penis length and girth. The results? Of the 170 women who were kind enough to fill out the questionnaire between nursing their newborn babies, 21 percent reported that they found the length of a guy's penis to be important, while 32 percent reported that girth is important. (Note that every woman who reported length as important also said girth was important.) The researchers concluded that a good percentage of women attach importance to the size of a guy's package.[52] What they didn't ask was whether these women preferred big over small or thick over thin.

And ladies, especially with the Hulk, lubrication is critical. Even if you are dripping wet, we suggest you supplement your natural juices with a healthy dollop of water-based lubrication.

THE TALL DRINK OF WATER

(At least 7 inches [17.8 centimeters] in length and 4 inches [10 centimeters] or thinner in circumference)

These long and slender guys can be a lot of fun to play with, as they are easy to wrap your hand or mouth around, and some women simply love the feel of a long cock inside of them. Just like Rhett Butler, played by the oh-so-drinkable Clark Gable in *Gone with the Wind*, these guys slide in nice and smooth. But as Scarlett O'Hara knows too well, if you don't handle them properly, they can leave you feeling pricked and stung. That's right, girls, due to the length of the Tall Drink of Water, intercourse brings the risk of painful cervix bumping.

Perfect Positions

Try the **Jockey (see pages 106-107)**: Start by lying either on your back or your stomach, with your legs spread open. Your guy straddles the outside of your legs and hips in a crouching position, much like that of a jockey (or a certain southern scoundrel we know and love—yum!) riding a racehorse. Let him gently enter you, and then, before he gets too excited and starts thrusting away, squeeze your legs closed around him. This position limits the depth of penetration so you can avoid any uncomfortable bumping sensations, and it also lets him feel fully enveloped because your thighs will press pleasingly around any parts of the shaft that don't make it inside your body. And if his penis is of the super slender variety, having your legs (and pussy) clamped tightly around his cock will provide the luscious sensation that he has additional girth.

Alternatively, ask him to be your **Bodyguard (see page 109)**. With both of you standing, have your guy enter you from behind. If there is a major height difference you (or he) may need to stand on a step or stool

(or you can put on your 6-inch stilettos) to attain the right fit. Because he's entering from behind without you being bent over, he can use his length to both of your advantage. Also, this frees up his hands to give you a breast or clit massage. You can reach behind and caress his buttocks
as he thrusts his way to bliss.

If his length isn't all that bothersome to you and you've been practicing yoga, ask him to do the **Pile Driver**. Ⓑ This is one super kinky position that guys of shorter endowments may have trouble accomplishing. In this position, lie on your upper back and raise your lower back and butt off the floor, completely exposing your pussy and pushing your booty skyward. Support your hips with your hands, elbows pressed into the floor. Your knees will fall to either side of your ears. Standing, he straddles you, bending his penis down toward the floor as he enters you. The thrusting motion comes from him squatting and standing as he penetrates. Now he can get to drilling!

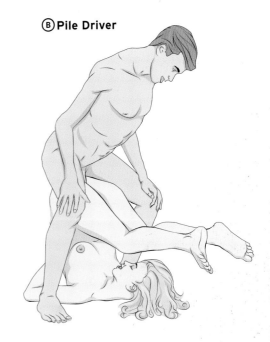
Ⓑ **Pile Driver**

Tasty Tips
If in any position you try, you find that your guy is so long that he uncomfortably pokes your cervix while thrusting, you can further control the depth of his insertion by wrapping your hand around the base of his penis and giving him a tight squeeze as you ride.

Practicing your Kegels (which you should do no matter what size your guy is) will help you to make the most of the Tall Drink of Water. Tone your vaginal muscles by repetitively squeezing and releasing them. One Kegel consists of both tightening and relaxing the muscle, so begin by tightening your pelvic muscle for three seconds, and relaxing for three seconds. Do ten reps, three times a day. As you get stronger, you can increase the contraction/relaxation time incrementally from three seconds up to ten seconds. The great thing about Kegels is, you can do your reps while sitting at your computer or driving, and nobody will be the wiser! During sex, this strength will help you get a grip around his penis. Doing Kegels also enhances your orgasms, as these are some of the same muscles that contract during your climax.

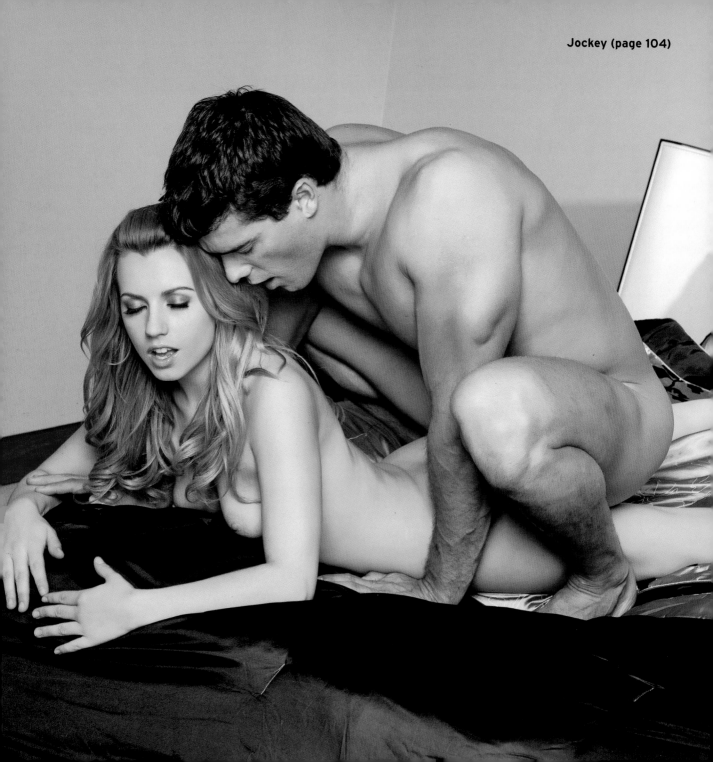

Jockey (page 104)

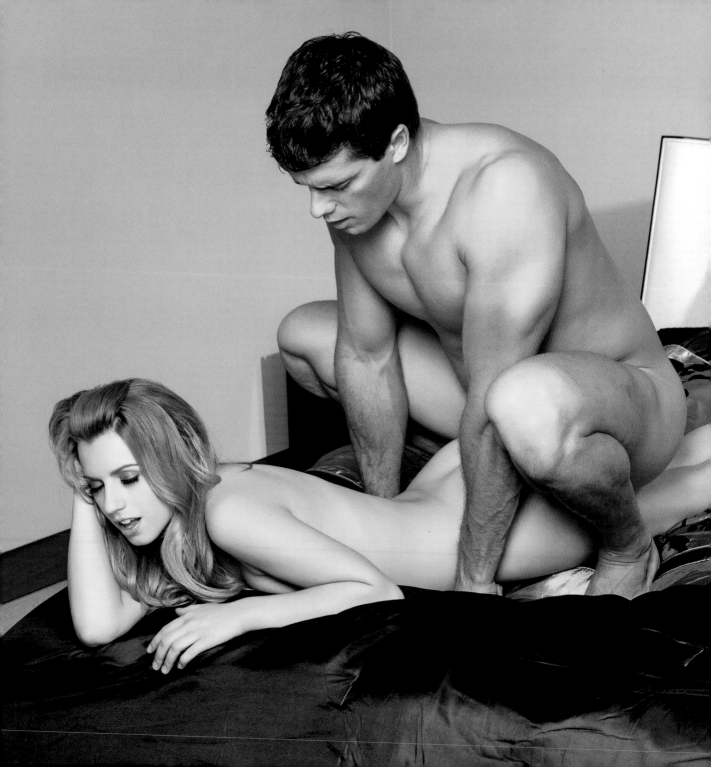

THE BUBBA

(6.5 inches [16.5 centimeters] or fewer in length and at least 5 inches [12.7 centimeters] in circumference)

The Bubba may be considered the perfect package for those women who love the sensation of being stretched open, yet prefer to have their cervixes left untouched. For yet others, the stretching part may still be a bit of a challenge to overcome.

Perfect Positions

Since controlling depth isn't the issue here, it's best to really open your legs wide for Bubba. The **Missionary** position, and many open-legged variations of Missionary, such as the **Pirate's Bounty** © (one leg stretched wide to the side, while the other rests on his shoulder), should provide for perfectly pleasurable penetration. Also, **Standing Doggy Style**, leaning forward over the bed (or your office desk) with your legs spread wide, is a good choice for playing with Bubba.

Tasty Tips

If your vagina is resistant to stretching wide, perform many of the same warm-up exercises described for preparing for the Hulk. Heck, it wouldn't hurt to insist that your guy give you a pre-penetration orgasm via tongue, finger, or toy every time. Just tell him you *couldn't possibly* handle his huge package without one. Buttering him up is the best way to get him to butter *you* up.

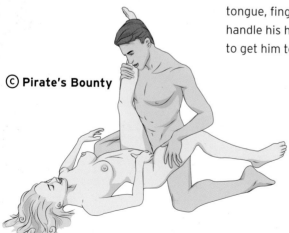

© Pirate's Bounty

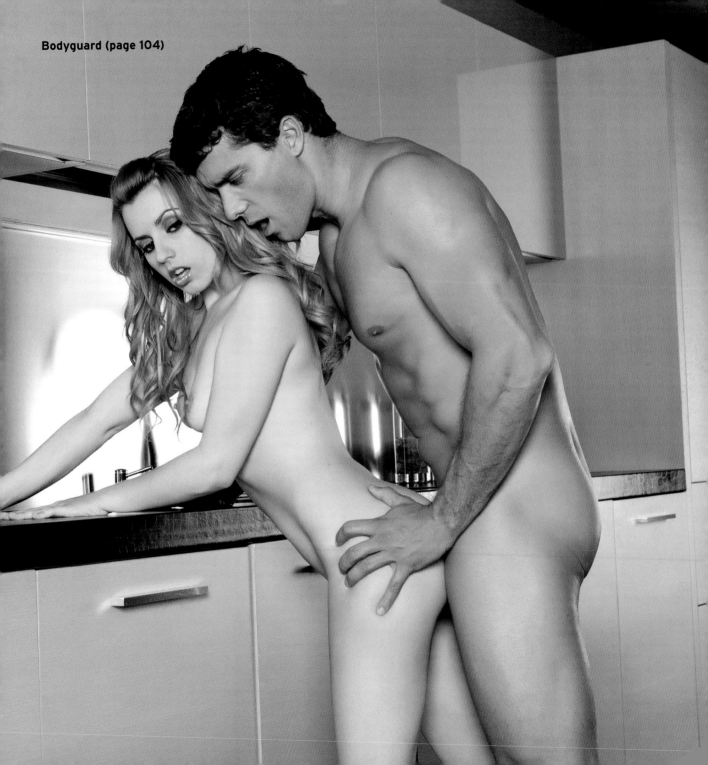

Bodyguard (page 104)

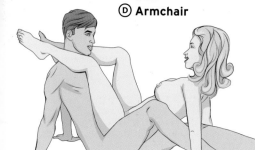

Ⓓ **Armchair**

MR. HAPPY

(5 to 6 inches [12.7 to 15.2 centimeters] in length and 4 to 5 inches [10.2 to 12.7 centimeters] in circumference)

Most women are more than happy to have a Mr. Happy to play with, as they are perfectly designed to fit snugly within the dimensions of the average woman's vagina. Typically, sexual encounters with these perfectly medium-sized guys leave little to worry about when it comes to trying a variety of sexual positions, because most of them will be a sure fit.

Perfect Positions

Any position is usually a good position with Mr. Happy, but here are a few fun ones you might not have tried before: If you've both been working on your triceps at the gym, try the **Armchair** position. Ⓓ Your guy sits beneath you on a flat surface with his legs extended while supporting his weight on his arms. You sit in his lap facing him and prop your legs up on his shoulders, leaning back, and supporting yourself by your arms. The motion comes from you using your arms to rock back and forth along his cock. This position provides a nice angle for hitting your G-spot.

For a less strenuous but just as sexy position, try the **Lap Dance (see page 111)**. Your man sits on a couch or chair, and you sit in his lap, facing away from him. Grind your way to a delightful climax.

Tasty Tips

One of the best things about Mr. Happy is that his average size makes him perfect for trying some extra-kinky moves and positions—one of our favorites being **Double Penetration**. Add a small- to medium-sized dildo to your sex play and try using it in your anus while Mr. Happy makes your pussy happy (or vice versa). This is a fun way to fulfill your fantasy of a threesome, without the potential jealousy headache. If you find that you like the sensation, be sure to invest in plenty of lube.

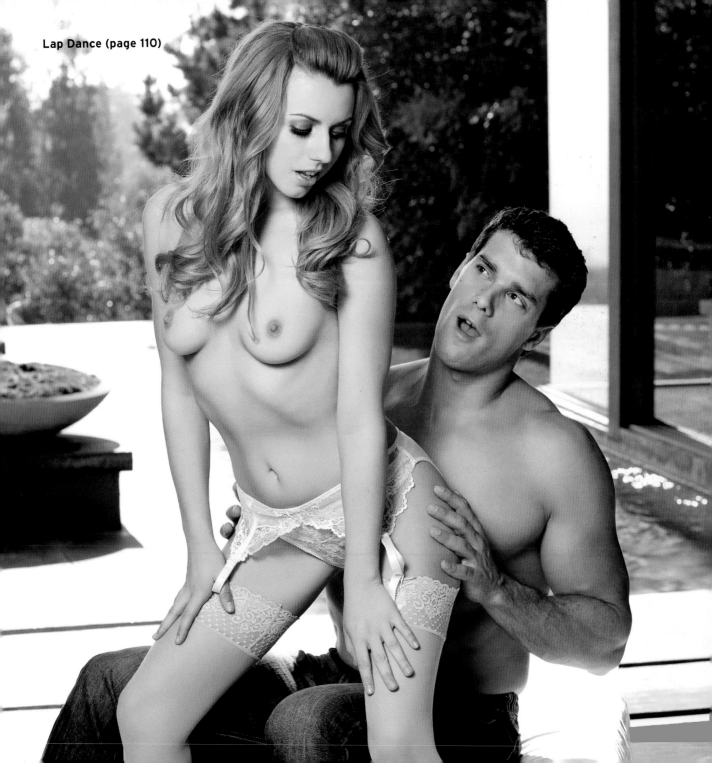

Lap Dance (page 110)

THE MAVERICK

(Less than 5 inches [12.7 centimeters] in length and 3.5 inches [8.9 centimeters] or less in circumference)

We call this cock Maverick because it's short and slender, à la Tom Cruise's sexy fighter pilot character in *Top Gun*. There is something quite delightful about finding this loveable lollipop in your guy's underpants. Sure, Maverick may not provide that stretched-to-the-brim feeling that some women love, but sex is about *so much more* than just feeling filled, and that's often where Maverick comes into play. As far as pleasure and true stimulation goes for women, it's only the first 3 inches (7.6 centimeters) of our vaginas that are sensitive to touch—anything deeper and all we feel is pressure. For tickling, teasing, and stroking these sensitive few inches, including the G-spot, Maverick is more than equipped to "buzz the tower" and bring you home to a landing pad of orgasms.

Perfect Positions

Doggy Style is the classic go-to position for mutual enjoyment with Maverick. The trick is positioning: Instead of resting on all fours, lower your arms and head to the bed, so that your ass is sticking up in the air. Arch your spine and draw your thighs together. When he goes in from behind at this angle, Maverick can feel quite large, and this is hands down one of the best positions for hitting your G-spot. As an added bonus, Maverick is one partner with whom Doggy Style will be pain-free—unless, of course, you beg for plenty of spankings to go along with the penetration.

   Bunny Ears Ⓔ is another position that's just perfect for your Maverick. Lie down on your back, spread your legs, and draw your knees up close to your ears. Have your lover place a pillow under your bottom,

Ⓔ **Bunny Ears**

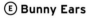

and he can also help hold your legs in position. Your pelvis will be tipped in such a way that it will feel like his cock is filling your entire pussy. And, interestingly, this is another great position for prime G-spot stimulation.

Don't overlook the potential pleasure of anal play. Maverick may be just the perfect toy to put in your pretty puckerhole; no pain, just fun. Of course, because Mother Nature didn't equip your booty with its own natural secretions, don't forget to add water-based lube! And last, Maverick may be one of the best penis sizes out there when it comes to giving head. You can suck, lick, tongue, and swallow to your heart's content without ever experiencing the discomfort of gagging or an assault on the back of your throat.

Tasty Tips

If you've already experienced a number of orgasms or heightened arousal beforehand, just the sensation of his hard penis brushing up against your sensitive clit and labia may be enough to send you over the edge. A man who owns a Maverick is usually an amazing lover because he masters how to pleasure a woman with more than just his cock. But if your Maverick hasn't aced his flight tests yet, why not play sexy flight instructor to this passionate, bad-boy pilot?

To give Maverick a temporary boost in the size department, try having him wear a cock ring (see chapter three), which can slightly amplify the size of his erection. Also, there is nothing better than incorporating your favorite vibrator into sex play.

THE ACROBAT

(A penis of any size that is bent at a significant angle— either right, left, up, or down)

The challenge with the Acrobat is finding a position that allows for comfortable entry. Happily, you might find that his particular angle can rub you in exactly the right way. (Note that if his bend is very extreme, it could be an indication that he has a medical condition called Peyronie's disease; see chapter nine for more information.)

SCIENTIFICALLY SPEAKING: WHAT IS A MICROPENIS?

A **micropenis** is a medical condition that affects less than one percent of all men. A micropenis is only one inch long when erect, usually accompanied by normal-sized testicles. The condition can be caused by a variety of congenital defects, the most common being prenatal androgen deficiency. A man with this condition may elect to surgically enlarge his penis using penile implants, although this procedure is yet to be perfected.[57]

> **The great thing about sex is that, when approached with a smile, it's the trials and errors as well as the orgasmic successes that make it fun!**

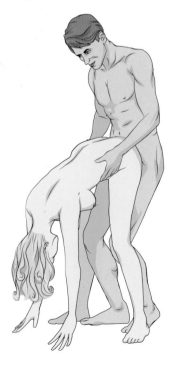

Ⓕ **Ben Dover**

Perfect Positions

Typically, you are going to want to position your body so that it complements his angle of entry. For example, a guy whose penis curves toward the floor may have better luck entering you from a rear-entry position, such as the **Ben Dover** Ⓕ. Start by standing, and then bend over so that your hands touch the floor with your butt pointed skyward. Your guy then penetrates you comfortably from behind. Note that if he's not much taller than you are, a kneeling Doggy Style position may work better.

Guys with a lefty bend may want to try **Spoons**, a position where you both lie on your right sides and he penetrates you from behind; for the guy with a righty bend, just flip it around and lie on your left sides.

A man whose penis curves up and points back toward his belly button may be able to find his path to paradise with you on top—and lucky for you this is often the best-shaped cock for rubbing your G-spot just right. Try the **Dirty Secretary (see page 115)**: Have him sit upright in an office chair and then straddle him, keeping your feet on the ground for the ultimate in thrusting control.

Tasty Tips

Just because you find one position that works best doesn't mean that you shouldn't explore other options. You'll find the more you explore, the more positions you'll discover that will allow his specially curved penis to rub you in just the right way. The great thing about sex is that, when approached with a smile, it's the trials and errors as well as the orgasmic successes that make it fun!

Remember, ladies, dicks come in a variety of shapes and sizes. We encourage you to get to know the unique plaything that he has hiding in his boxers and make the most of it! Take your time and have fun examining and exploring the many ways his unique penis proportions can pleasure you. This is all an important part of becoming a true penis genius.

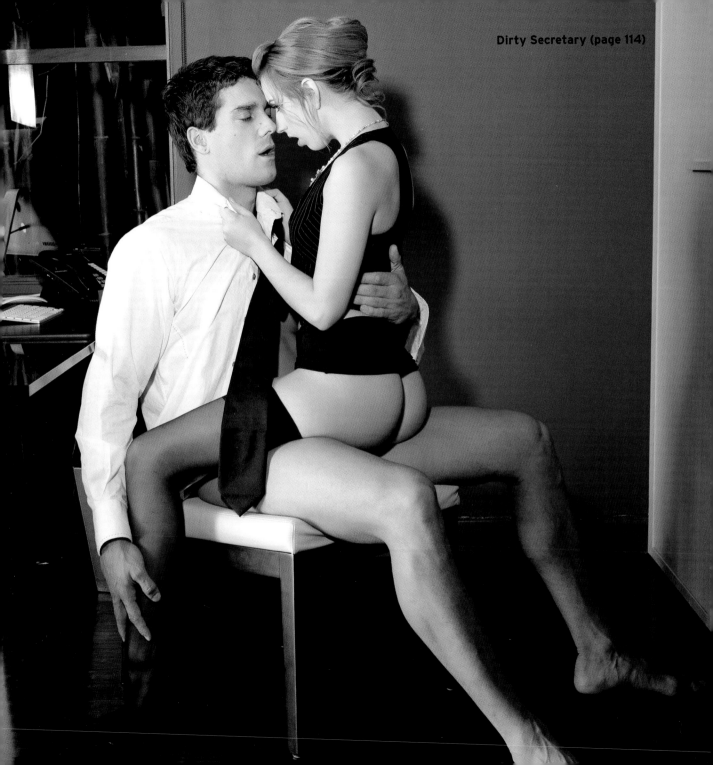

Dirty Secretary (page 114)

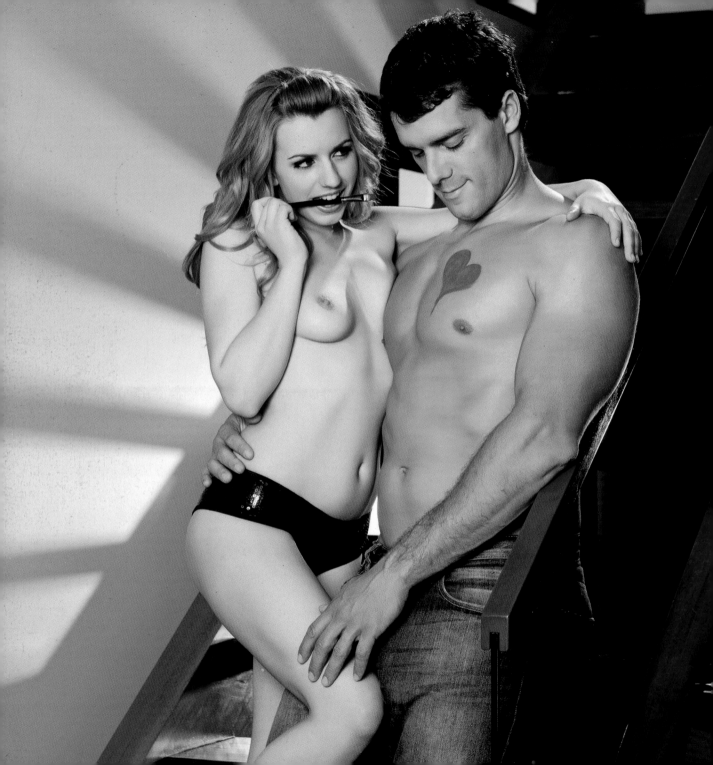

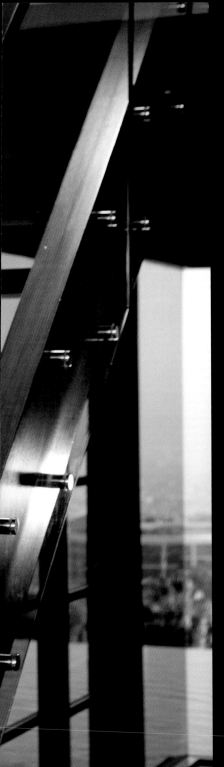

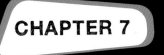

CHAPTER 7

PENILE ALTERATIONS: FASCINATING, BUT NOT FOR THE FAINT OF HEART

Although circumcision is the most widely practiced male genital modification, there are quite a few other ways to change the appearance of his phallus. From piercings and tattoos to phalloplasty (surgical penis enlargement), men have been decorating and altering their penises for thousands of years.

In the 1800s, it was the fashion for men to wear tight, white pants. To avoid an obvious bulge in their trousers, historical rumor has it that they wore a ring in the head of their penises that attached to a hook inside their pant leg.

Raven Rowanchild of the Department of Sociology at the University of Toronto postulates, "Extreme male genital modifications not only honestly advertise status, sexual potency, and ability to provide sexual satisfaction, they may provide a reliable index of male-female cooperation through the male's commitment to endure pain and risk."[58] What she's trying to say is this: Some women get turned on by a guy who's not afraid to poke a needle in his junk!

PENIS PIERCING

Today, the practice of male genital piercing is popular among men of a daring sexual nature. Piercing is often viewed as both a form of adornment and a way to erotically stimulate a man and his partner. There are more types of genital piercing than there is room to describe them in this book, so let's investigate some of the more well-known variations.

Prince Albert

One of the most common male genital piercings, the Prince Albert (PA) is named after Prince Albert (1819–1861) of Saxe-Coburg and Gotha, husband to his first cousin Queen Victoria of the United Kingdom of Great Britain and Ireland. Prince Albert wasn't a rebel; in fact, he was an upstanding politician who, among other projects, worked hard for the abolishment of slavery. One popular but unverified story behind the PA is that the prince was merely following the trends of the time. In the 1800s, it was the fashion for men to wear tight, white pants. To avoid an obvious bulge in their trousers, historical rumor has it that they wore a ring in the head of their penises that attached to a hook inside their pant leg. Tailors asked men if they dressed left or dressed right (meaning, did their penis hang naturally to the right, or to the left?). They then placed the hook in the corresponding leg of their pants.[59] Men today are still asked whether they dress left or right, but typically forego the piercing and hook.

The Prince Albert piercing is threaded through the urethra opening in the head of the penis and out just to the side of the frenulum. With the emerging popularity of skinny jeans, perhaps the piercing will gain the popularity it once had in the nineteenth century, but for now, it's considered quite a novelty.

Frenum Piercing

In an 1884 ethnology publication, it was noted that the Timorese of Indonesia pierced their frenula with brass rings in a quest for enhanced sexual stimulation.[60] Today, this piercing is popular among the sexually adventurous for the same reason. A barbell or a small ring is threaded from one side to the other through the frenulum, just under the head of a man's penis. An even more extreme variation of this piercing is known as the "frenum ladder," where a series of barbells are pierced along the underside of his cock, starting at the frenulum and going all the way to the top of his scrotum. Says twenty-eight-year-old Samuel about his frenum ladder, "I have had sex with two girls since getting my jewelry. Both women said it was the best experience they have ever had because the texture felt really good. For me, besides pleasing my girl, sometimes the piercing creates a pinching sensation that feels good."

Foreskin Piercing (Infibulation)

In ancient Greece, athletes performed nude. How's an athlete to prevent his penis from flopping around in the wind, then? Tie his foreskin to the base of his dick with a leather ribbon, of course! This technique is said to have led to infibulation, a method wherein the foreskin is pierced and then fastened to a second piercing on the scrotum or perineum (a perineum piercing is known as a guiche). If a man is lacking a foreskin, the Prince Albert piercing can be used in the same manner. Aside from keeping the penis secure and flop-free, infibulation also prevents erections, because it prevents adequate blood flow to the penis. The Romans are said to have used this method to enforce abstinence in their slaves, and today it has become a practice among some of those in the BDSM (bondage, domination, submission/sadomasochism) lifestyle as a way to erotically control a partner.[61]

 FAMOUS PENIS: ELMO-THE-PENIS

The Icelandic Phallological Museum in Húsavík is home to 271 (and growing) specimens of mammalian penises. Amid its collection will soon reside Elmo-the-Penis, to be donated by American Stan Underwood while he is still living(!). His penis is impressive in size and has a tattoo of a heart on its head (although rumors have it that he'll be covering the heart up with a more patriotic American Eagle before donating his dick). In commentary written by "Elmo" for humanpenis.org, the decision is explained: "He [Underwood] would really like to witness my removal from his body, and placement as a separate entity in a place where I can be shown with honor and dignity." As of publication, Underwood is waiting for a sponsor to help him cover the cost of the expensive surgery to remove his penis from his body.[66, 67]

IMPORTANT TIPS FOR HEALTHY PENIS PIERCING

1. Choose a studio with a good reputation that specializes in body piercing.

2. Be sure the studio uses the autoclave method to sterilize the piercing equipment. Needles should be single-use only, so it should come fresh out of the package and be carefully disposed of after use. If the piercing artist pulls a needle out of a jar of disinfectant, run and don't look back!

3. Follow all aftercare instructions. This will include abstaining from sex (yes, this includes oral sex) for about six weeks, using antiseptics (e.g., Bactine) and salt-water solutions, and handling the penis with clean hands.

4. After the piercing is fully healed, keeping it clean is still important. Be sure to wash regularly with soap and water. If you ever notice any pus or irritation in the piercing, remove the jewelry immediately. If it doesn't clear up in a few days, or if he develops a fever or rash, have him seek medical attention.

Apadravya Piercing

This piercing goes vertically from the upper side of the glans to the underside, passing through the urethra. It finds its roots in the Kama Sutra, which says, "He should pierce the lingam with a very sharp instrument and then sit in water until the bleeding has stopped. The same evening he should indulge in a very active form of sexual intercourse so that the hole can be cleansed." The book then goes on to suggest that a man can fill the hole with things like a wooden mortar or a heron's bone, all in the name of sexual enhancement.[62]

Today a man will be advised to not engage in any sexual activity for several weeks after receiving a piercing, and he'll probably be advised to wear stainless steel jewelry and not to insert wood or bones into his piercing hole—but the general principal remains the same. The piercing is meant to be a source of erotic pleasure for both the man and his partner.

GENITAL TATTOOS

The decision to tattoo one's penis is usually borne of a tremendous fondness for both tattoos and pain. But some men get them as a handy excuse to pull their dicks out of their pants. In *The Book of the Penis*, Maggie Paley writes, "Mad Dog, a famous San Francisco tattoo artist, told me he'd tattooed the words 'your name' on the penis of one of his customers. This man wanted it so he could go into a bar and say to whomever he pleased, 'I'll bet you I have your name tattooed on my dick.'"[63] What a clever pick-up line (or way to win bets)!

Although the practice isn't popular in the mainstream, many a brave body-art connoisseur has opted to decorate his rod with ink. One example is alternative porn star Rob Rotten, who among his many other body tattoos, has the word *poison* tattooed along the upper side of his shaft. (We just hope he's not trying to warn women of some kind of sexually transmitted infection he might be carrying.)

Rotten is hardly the first guy to get his shaft decorated. A Scythian chieftain mummy, dated to about 500 to 300 BC and unearthed in Siberia in 1947, was heavily tattooed from torso to penis.[64] Another example is in early Samoan culture; men were given full-body tattoos in order to achieve the title of *matai* (or chief). This included tattooing the anus, perineum, scrotum, and penis.[65]

Not every tattoo artist is willing to give a modern man a colorful penis, so if your man is looking to get decorated, he should call around to various shops first. It's also best to find an artist who has previous experience putting needles to wieners. You hardly want to be the first penis the tattoo artist has decorated! Many artists, but not all, will charge a handling fee in addition to their regular tattooing fee, simply because handling a guy's dick isn't their favorite thing to do. In addition, because the skin on the penis is malleable, the tattooist may warn you that over time the ink of the tattoo will fade or bleed out. And don't worry about putting him on Viagra or getting a fluffer to accompany him to the parlor; typically a tattoo is performed on a flaccid penis that is stretched out, as it's difficult for men to maintain an erection while in pain.

Men who've gotten penis tattoos report that they were no more painful than being tattooed elsewhere on the body. Says twentysomething Phil, "For me, any pain is overshadowed by the sense of pleasure and enjoyment that I get from having a decorated penis. Basically, for the most part, it does not hurt any more than any other kind of tattoo."

PENIS ENLARGEMENT

Men's obsession with penis size has caused some of them to go to extreme measures in an effort to alter the appearance of their dicks. Hanging weights, jelqing, and surgery are just a few of the methods that men have tested in their quest for the perfectly sized penis.

Hanging Weights

Internet rumor has it that hanging weights off one's penis will naturally enlarge it. Sites backing this rumor usually refer to men of the Ugandan Karamojong tribe (who are purported to have exceptionally large penises), saying that they have used hanging penis weights for thousands of years. Most often, these sites invoke such rumors to encourage people to buy specialized penis weights or other enlargement products.

IMPORTANT TIPS FOR HEALTHY PENIS TATTOOING

1. Do your research and find a reputable tattoo studio with an artist experienced in genital tattoos.

2. Be sure the studio uses the autoclave method to sterilize its equipment. The tattoo artist should also pour ink into single-serving cups just for you (so he or she doesn't double dip into ink that's been used on someone else).

3. Abstain from sex for about two weeks, or until the tattoo is fully healed.

4. Keep your tat clean and use antibacterial or protective ointments as suggested by the artist (a favorite is Aquaphor by Eucerin).

5. Avoid wearing tight pants (or any pants at all) for a few days, because contact with clothing can irritate the freshly wounded skin.

> If the Karamojong penis size is long enough to capture the attention of those selling penis enlargement equipment and techniques, it has to do with their genes and not hanging circular stone disks on the tips of their penises.

Love Doctor Yangki Christine Akiteng, a native Ugandan, writes that, although Karamojong men indeed have penises that hang to about mid thigh (and they traditionally don't wear pants), they do not use hanging weights. She says, "If the Karamojong penis size is long enough to capture the attention of those selling penis enlargement equipment and techniques, it has to do with their genes and not hanging circular stone disks on the tips of their penises. If you don't believe me, take a trip to Karamoja and see if you see any boys with stones or discs hanging on the tips of their penises. I am even happy to accompany you, provided you pay for my airfare."[68] Additionally, people who have tried this "ancient" technique have reported problems such as burst blood vessels, scarring, nerve damage, and impotence. Simply put: It doesn't work, and it may even permanently damage your package!

Jelqing

Another widespread Internet rumor claims that jelqing, an all-natural exercise, can increase penis size. The procedure, said to be Arabic in origin, takes thirty minutes per day and involves stroking the penis in a specific way. There is talk of a study by Dr. Brian Richards in the 1970s that supports the exercise's effectiveness (although Richards calls it the Chartham method), but the original article is never referenced.[69] In fact, most of the articles that describe this exercise also offer tools for sale that are said to make jelqing easier. Reputable science journals make no mention of jelqing except to mention that it is a bogus method that can cause damage to the penis. Christopher Wanjek, writing for LiveScience.com, says, "[Jelqing] makes no sense biologically, however, and one runs the risk of tearing blood vessels and losing sensitivity if one tugs too hard for too long. Those thirty minutes could be spent doing sit-ups for sexier results."[70]

Phalloplasty

Experts agree that surgery is the only tested and effective method to enlarge a man's penis. But it doesn't come without risks or the chance of complications.

For thousands of dollars, a man can opt to gain about an inch to his ding-dong via a surgical lengthening procedure. The surgery involves cutting one of the two ligaments that suspends the penis, allowing the root of the penis (which is inside his body) to drop an additional 1 to 1.5 inches (2.5 to 3.8 centimeters) from the body. It's not really an addition—after surgery, more of his penis is exposed than before. Sadly, side effects can include depression, numbness, and impotence, and even if all goes well, without that ligament intact, his erection may start to look a little droopy.

Men can also opt to have girth added to their dicks via a couple of methods. The first is a fat transfer. The doctor uses liposuction to collect fat from his belly or thighs and then injects it into the penile shaft just beneath the surface of the skin. Unfortunately, over time the girth is lost as the body reabsorbs the fat cells. And sometimes the fat redistributes itself and gives the penis a lumpy appearance.

The second technique for adding girth is called a dermal-fat graft, during which large grafts of all seven layers of skin (including dermal fat) are transferred from the thighs to the penis and layered on top like a birthday cake (or more aptly, an onion). If a man doesn't want to use his own skin (which is invasive, painful, and may cause scarring), he can opt to use skin from a deceased donor. One of the latest techniques developed by LifeCell Corporation uses a substance called AlloDerm. In this procedure, strips of freeze-dried skin taken from cadavers are layered over the top of the penis, much like in a regular dermal-fat graft procedure.

Although experts seem to agree that surgery is most likely a man's best bet for penis enlargement, the American Urological Association supports neither the lengthening methods nor the fat injection methods (the jury is still out on fat grafting). The association says that these procedures have "not been shown to be safe or efficacious."[71]

Whether your man chooses to embellish his penis with jewels or colors or tries to change its shape or size is really up to him. We think most women would agree: We'd take a healthy, natural, small or average cock over an altered penis any day. What you can do is encourage him to love his body the way it is and let him know that the sexiest adornment is you.

> The second technique for adding girth is called a dermal-fat graft, during which large grafts of all seven layers of skin (including dermal fat) are transferred from the thighs to the penis and layered on top like a birthday cake (or more aptly, an onion).

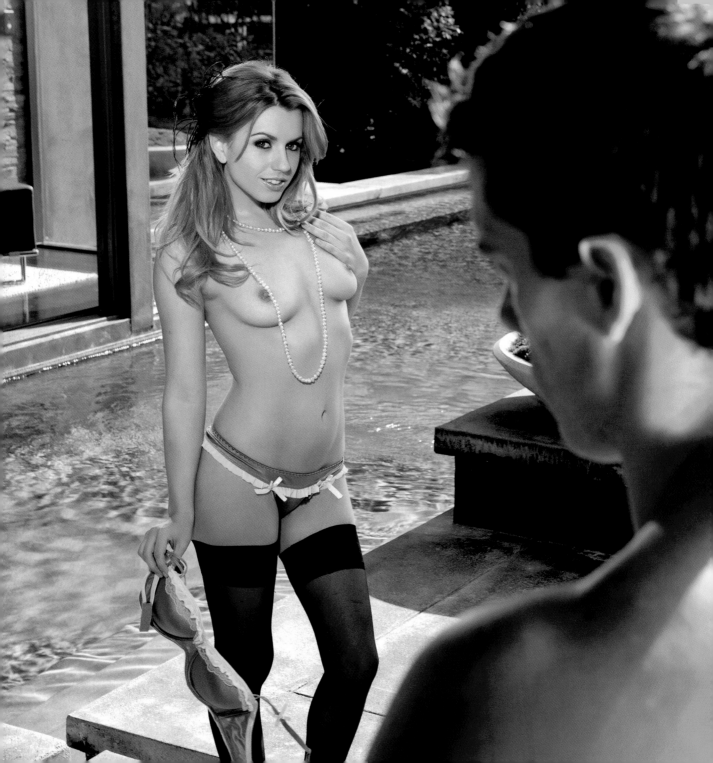

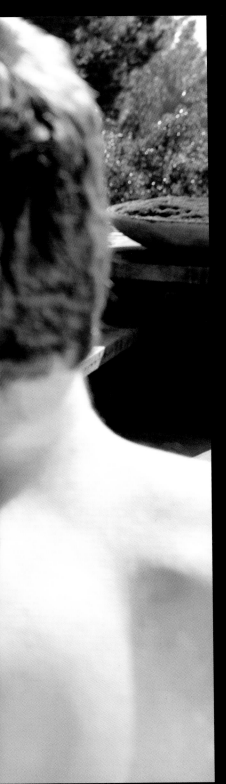

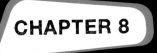

CHAPTER 8

THE PENIS SHRINK: WHAT MAKES HIS OTHER HEAD TICK?

What makes that little head tick? In this chapter, we'll explore different ways his brain and other senses affect the function of his cock. We'll also touch on some of the weirder and funnier manifestations of the human psyche as it relates to the penis.

THE EYE-TO-COCK CONNECTION

It's taken for granted that men are visual creatures, and it could be argued that there is a direct connection between his eyes and his cock. Research scientists agree that a man experiences visual stimuli differently than women. In a study by Stephan Hamann et al. of Emory University, both men and women were subjected to fMRIs (functional magnetic resonance imaging) to monitor brain activity while they were exposed to erotic imagery. Researchers found that the amygdala (which is linked to emotions, aggression, and sexual arousal) and hypothalamus (responsible for regulating metabolic processes, among other things) are more strongly activated in men than in women when viewing identical sexual stimuli.[72]

Why not use his sense of sight to your advantage? Knowing that you are visually stimulating your partner can be an incredible turn-on for you as well. Following are some sexy ideas.

Do It with the Lights On

Yup, it's that simple! In our survey, we found that 82.5 percent of men prefer sex with the lights on, and 79 percent say they get off more easily when they can see what's happening. This doesn't mean that you have to set up hot stage lights in your bedroom (unless you want to put on a homemade porn production . . . which could be fun). Lord knows that sometimes having the lights turned up makes us a bit self-conscious about whatever we imagine we have to be worried about. (Really, a little cellulite won't send your husband running for the hills, we swear!) There are ways to use your man's wish to see you in the light to get you both in the mood, without lighting up your perceived flaws in the process. Here are a few sexy ways to turn the lights (and him) on:

❶ Early morning light is soft and sexy. Before the sun has risen all the way, open the curtains and let the soft light enhance your lovemaking. Not into first-thing-in-the-morning sex? Get up half an hour early, pee, and brush your teeth, and maybe enjoy a cup of coffee first.

2. Holiday lights work their magic all year long. Try stringing up a set of white holiday lights around your bedroom, your living room, or even your back patio, wherever you want to feel seductive. Says thirtysomething Phil, "I love to watch my penis enter her—the combination of the sensation of pushing into her and the visual of watching it happen is absolutely incredible! I also love to watch her facial expressions and body's reaction as she builds towards orgasm."

3. Use a few flickering candles to set the mood. After a romantic meal at home, set the evening on fire with a blazing candelabra and a little sexy lovemaking on the dining room table for dessert. Just don't knock the candles over—even though firemen are sexy, a burning dining room set will ruin the mood.

4. Lay out a blanket in front of your lit fireplace. The crackling wood, dancing light, and warmth will generate hot passion. Says fortysomething Jeremy, "The shadows of light reflecting off her breasts and outlining her curves are incredibly sensuous! She is a visual delight!"

5. Use nightlights, ambient light, or a dimly lit doorway for a small amount of light (without the pressure of full-on, 100-watt light bulbs).

Play Dress Up

Men love lingerie. Matching sets of lace undergarments, negligees, and corsets with garters and high-heeled shoes are a few of the fun items you can wear. Says fortysomething Barnabus, "Ahhh, the thought of long limbs and luscious curves in sexy garments is enough to feed any man's imagination and libido." Don't worry if your expensive silk and lace ends up on the floor more quickly than you had anticipated. That doesn't mean that the lingerie didn't work. Your body in seductive garments simply makes him want to see you entirely naked all the more quickly.

Seventy-nine percent say they get off more easily when they can see what's happening. This doesn't mean that you have to set up hot stage lights in your bedroom (unless you want to put on a homemade porn production . . . which could be fun).

You don't have to take out stock in Victoria's Secret to get the desired effect. Wear your man's T-shirt with nothing underneath, or try a pair of his underwear with nothing on top.

Remember that you don't have to save your lingerie for the bedroom; you can wear it around the house on a lazy Sunday afternoon or wear it while you cook a romantic dinner. Says fiftysomething Bob, "There is nothing more exciting than to see her do something mundane in her sexy get-ups, like when she does the dishes in a teddy and heels."

Also note that you don't have to take out stock in Victoria's Secret to get the desired effect. Wear your man's T-shirt with nothing underneath, or try a pair of his underwear with nothing on top. Says twentysomething Randy, "It's simple, but I like it when my girlfriend gets out of the shower and dries her hair wearing nothing but a towel."

Looking for a way to showcase all your sexiness? Try putting on a fashion show with your favorite lingerie, heels, or creative outfits of your own making. A scarf tied tightly across your breasts topped by a long jacket provides an alluring silhouette for him to admire!

The Art of Tasteful Flashing

Add a little danger and intrigue to your sex life by carefully flashing your man in unexpected places. The trick is to make sure he is the only one who sees your delectable parts. To make it easy, wear a skirt with nothing underneath. Try discreetly spreading your legs as you take your seat across from him at a dinner party, or briefly flip up the back of your skirt as he trails behind you at the market. Once he realizes you're wearing no panties, he'll lose his mind. Says Charles, a fortysomething attorney, "The sexiest thing my wife does is surprise me by showing me her pussy in a public place."

Have Sex in Front of a Mirror

Double your pleasure by allowing him to enjoy your mirror image while in the throes of passion. Says thirty-seven-year-old Carl, "We have had the opportunity a couple of times to have intercourse in front of a mirror or reflecting window, and we both enjoy watching our bodies' reactions, the penetration, and the fucking." Bend over the bathroom sink so he can get a nice image of your face and breasts in the mirror while he simultaneously enjoys the view of your backside. Mirrored headboards,

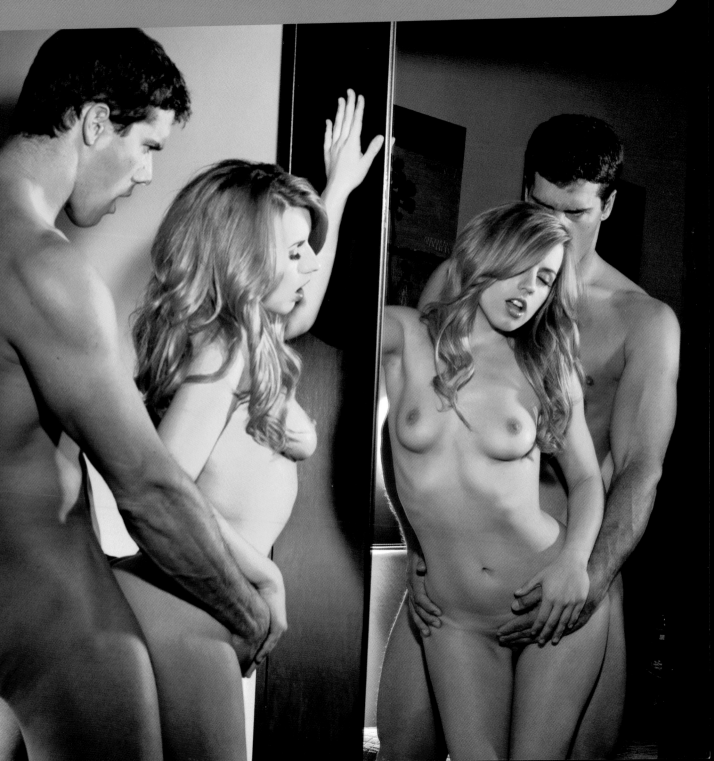

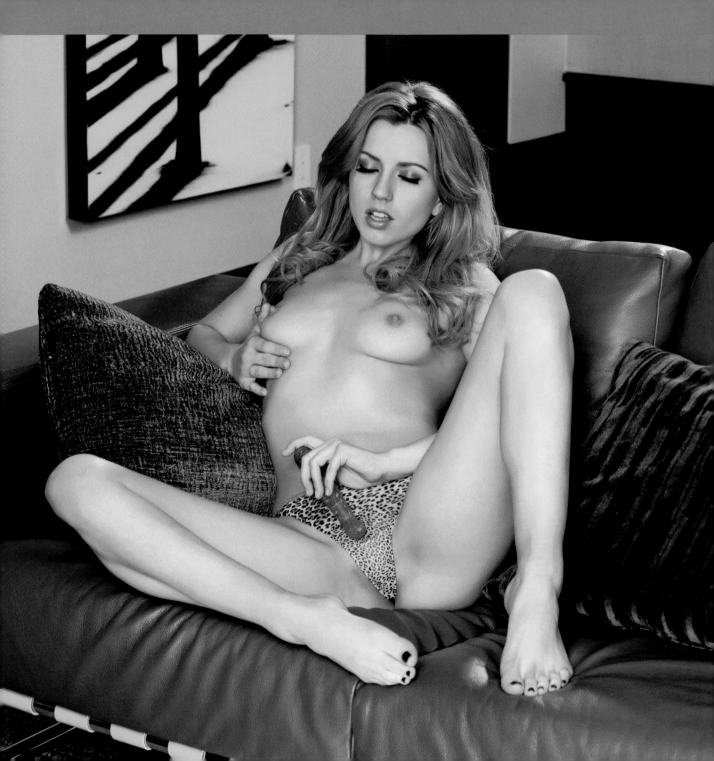

ceilings, and closet doors can also offer a delightful visual treat. For a super-dirty twist, when you're on all fours in Doggy Style, use a hand mirror to show him the view from beneath your body.

Masturbate for Him

When we asked our men what the sexiest thing a woman has ever done to visually stimulate them, far and away the most common response was that their lovers masturbated for them. If you feel shy, get yourself in the mood by warming up before the show. Here are some ideas:

1. Start masturbating before he comes in the room and let him "catch you" in the act.

2. Ask him to give you a little oral sex first to get you in the proper state of mind.

3. Wear a blindfold so you can completely close him out and just allow yourself to let go.

4. Watch him masturbate for you while you play with yourself for him.

5. Don't be afraid to add your favorite sex toy. Says fiftysomething Christopher, "The sexiest thing my wife ever did for me was let me watch as she masturbated with her dildo."

Anything that will bring you to orgasm will make the experience that much more exciting . . . for the both of you!

Sexy Photos and Films

Titillate your man by taking sexy photos of yourself or filming the two of you together so you can watch later. Your man will appreciate being able to relive your sexiness when you're not around. Moreover, the act of taking photos or videos during sex adds elements of exhibitionism and voyeurism that can be incredibly arousing for both parties. Says twentysomething Ray, "The sexiest thing my girlfriend does for me is to send erotic videos to my phone when I'm least expecting it."

SCIENTIFICALLY SPEAKING: MEN LIKE TO WATCH YOUR FACE DURING SEX

According to our survey, 32 percent of men reported that they love to look at your face during sex. This is backed by a 2004 study in which researchers subjected both men and women to erotic images and monitored their attentions by employing eye-tracking technology. Heather Rupp, Ph.D., of the Kinsey Institute reported, "Men looked at the female face much more than women, and both looked at the genitals comparably."[73]

What part of your partner's body do you best like to look at during sex?

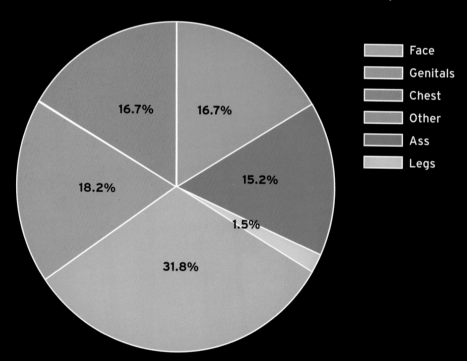

- Face
- Genitals
- Chest
- Other
- Ass
- Legs

16.7% 16.7% 15.2% 18.2% 1.5% 31.8%

The majority of men we surveyed like to watch a woman's face during sex, but your genitals and breasts also rank high.

A word of warning: Be aware in this day and age of the rapid sharing of information. It's best if you only share photos with someone who you completely trust and remove any identifying features from anything you send over the Internet or by cell phone. Better yet, use old school technology such as VHS recorders or Polaroid cameras so that you can easily keep track of your sexy images. And if you are a high-profile politician who could risk losing your career (yes, we're talking to YOU, John Edwards), it's probably best to not partake in this type of activity at all.

STRESSED OUT!

Stress can be a big factor in your guy's brain-to-penis connection. Of the men we surveyed, 60 percent reported that stress negatively affects their desire for sex. "When stressed, I can't even think about sex," says fortysomething Arnold.

Dr. Maryrose Gerardi of Emory University explains that the reason stress can cause a decrease in desire is simply because of fatigue. People who work over forty-eight hours per week or who don't get enough sleep often will lose their sex drive.[74]

Tips for Destressing Your Man

If your man's flagpole is at half-mast thanks to stress, here are some ideas to help him slow down and reconnect:

1. Give him an erotic massage. Not only are massages inherently relaxing, but they are sensual and can lead to sex. (For tips on giving a massage, read chapter four).

2. Have a sexy Sunday. Encourage him to sleep in, fix him breakfast in bed, and relax with a movie marathon interspersed with blow jobs, sex, and lots of snuggles.

3. Take a vacation. Even if it's just for a weekend, a change of scenery can do wonders for stress levels. Don't forget to pack a bag full of lingerie and sex toys.

> People who work over forty-eight hours per week or who don't get enough sleep often will lose their sex drive.[74]

SCIENTIFICALLY SPEAKING: SEX AND HIS SENSE OF SMELL

A study done in the 1990s suggests that smell combinations will get your man going. Dr. Alan R. Hirsch and his team conducted an experiment in which they subjected men to certain odor combinations and measured increases in penile blood flow. The most stimulating smells for the test subjects were the following:

- Lavender and pumpkin pie: 40 percent increase in penile blood flow
- Doughnuts and black licorice: 31.5 percent increase in penile blood flow
- Pumpkin pie and doughnuts: 20 percent increase in penile blood flow
- Orange: 19.5 percent increase in penile blood flow[75]

The conclusion? Men may be more aroused than we know when we're cooking up strange combinations of sweet treats!

On the flip side, sex can be a great way to relieve stress, and sometimes people turn to sex as a release when everything around them seems to be falling apart. In fact, 34 percent of the men we surveyed say that sometimes stress has the opposite effect and makes them want more sex. Trey, a fortysomething health regulator, says, "When I'm under pressure at work, it makes me horny and therefore sex is more intense and enjoyable." If you have one of these stress-loving studs, more power to you!

CHEATING BASTARDS

According to the University of Chicago's General Social Survey (GSS) that spanned the course of eleven years, researchers found that men are about twice as likely as women to cheat on their spouses. Five percent of men and 2.5 percent of women reported infidelity during a twelve-month time frame with their current spouse. Twenty-two percent of men and 12 percent of women reported having ever cheated in their lives.[76]

While our survey sample size was smaller and included nonmarried men, 43 percent of them admitted to having cheated. What's more, 76 percent of these guys said that cheating did *not* affect their ability to perform with their primary partners. Says twentysomething fast-food manager Len, "The girls I have gone steady with get my best. It's very easy for me to get fully hard with a person [who] I really care about even if I just fucked three other women." David, a thirtysomething teacher explains, "I was able to box up the two separate interactions in my mind and keep them apart."

A minority of men did report that the cheating affected their partnerships. Says Tim, a fortysomething Web developer, "I cheated online, and yes, the guilt impacted my performance with my wife."

Renowned biological anthropologist Dr. Helen Fisher explains to Discovery News why some people are able to cheat: "We've evolved three distinct brain systems for mating and reproduction. One is a sex drive, one is romantic love, and the third brain system is for attachment. . . . And these three brain systems aren't always well connected. You can feel deep attachment for one person, while you feel intense romantic love for someone else, while you feel the sex drive for a host of other individuals . . . the brain is built to enable us to love more than one person at a time. This is not to say that biology is destiny; we have an enormous cerebral cortex with which we make decisions . . . you can say no to adultery."[77]

PENIS ENVY

In the early 1900s, Sigmund Freud founded the basis for psychoanalysis and established major theories about how the mind develops and works. While much of his work is at the root of modern analysis and therapy, some of his theories have come under intense scrutiny. Freud had a certain special affection for the penis and placed such great importance on it that he theorized that all of basic human development is inextricably linked to the desire to own a penis. As part of his theory, he wrote that women experience "penis envy." As modern women, we have to wonder how much clout this idea of penis envy really has. Do women wish to have penises, or do they only wish that they could write their names in the snow? And on the flip side, do men ever wish they could have a vagina to call their own?

We discovered that, if anything, grown women experience "penis curiosity." That is, they'd like to have the opportunity to try one out for a day, but they are perfectly happy being endowed with what they were born with. Says thirty-six-year-old Ashley, "Being able to have a dick for a day would mean having permission to be wild and uninhibited without society thinking bad of me."

Says fortysomething Crystal, "When I was younger I was so envious of men who seemed to be able to come every time they had sex, and I wasn't coming at all. I thought it would be so cool to have the equipment to get off every time. . . . Once I found the right partners and learned about my own body, this wasn't so much a fantasy anymore . . . but I would like to feel what a man feels when he comes, or what it feels like to have a dick in a pussy. I don't want to be a man; I like my breasts too much . . . but for a day, it could be a lot of fun."

PENIS PANIC

Although we may panic about the swine flu and SARS, other cultures have been subjected to a different kind of panic. Penis panic (scientifically known as genital retraction syndrome) is a mass cultural belief that one's penis is actually retracting and will soon disappear. Penis panic has occurred in various populations in Asia and Africa. It's typically a method for people in positions of power to take control over a population by insinuating the imminent threat of the loss of a man's prized prowess. In 2001, an outbreak of penis panic occurred in the West African country of Benin, causing mobs to light innocent people on fire. The BBC reported, "The belief that men's private parts can mysteriously disappear through a handshake or an incantation is commonplace in Benin, where superstition and illiteracy are rife."[80]

We women have it all—breasts, vaginas, the ability to give birth . . . what do men have? Something that hangs out of the front of their pants that they give names to, for Chrissake!

Other women seemed rather appalled by the idea. Says thirtysomething Kris, "Have a penis? Absolutely not! While I adore penises on the opposite sex, I have never in my life wanted to have one (or experience being a man, for that matter). We women have it all—breasts, vaginas, the ability to give birth . . . what do men have? Something that hangs out of the front of their pants that they give names to, for Chrissake! And it doesn't always work all the time, either."

Twentysomething Gracie tells us matter-of-factly, "No, I don't want to have a penis—I just figure I can borrow one whenever I want and don't have to worry about maintenance and upkeep."

As it turns out, while most men are perfectly content with the equipment they were born with, some men experience a bit of "vagina curiosity." Says fortysomething Billy, "I told my wife if I had a pussy I would fuck myself to death, and she said, 'If you had a pussy you wouldn't think like that.'"

Fiftysomething Fred says, "I think most women would like to know what it feels like to be on the other end of a penis . . . just as I think most men would like to know what it feels like to be at the other end of a vagina. I know I would."

Thirty-eight-year-old Mac says, "I have often wondered what it would be like to have a vagina. What it actually feels like to have someone inside you and if it feels any different than being inside someone. My penis has its more sensitive areas, and I know what parts of my wife's vagina are most easily stimulated. So we are obviously similar, but what does it truly feel like?"

And when asked whether they thought women experienced penis envy, most of our gents suggested that women think the only advantage would be the ability to pee in public. Says twenty-three-year-old Jimmy, "They wish they could piss more conveniently when out in public." And twentysomething Tony quips, "No, she doesn't have penis envy . . . I mean, unless we're camping."

For those individuals who wish to experience what it's like to exist in the opposite gender's body, that may be a possibility someday. In the June 2010 *Science News*, researchers described a new experiment conducted via virtual reality. Cognitive scientist Mel Slater of University of Barcelona explains, "Guys who spend time looking at a simulated world through a life-size virtual girl's eyes feel as if they reside in her body." They also reported that the illusion persisted even when the perspective changed from first person to the men looking at the girl from third person. The men still felt like they were playing the part of the girl.[79] While this isn't quite the same as experiencing the opposite sex's genitalia, it's one step closer.

SCIENTIFICALLY SPEAKING: WHAT DO HORMONES HAVE TO DO WITH CHEATING?

It appears that Mother Nature wasn't quite sure what she wanted to do with the human race when it came to wiring us for monogamy or promiscuity. On the one hand, scientists say that the shape of the penis and large size of the testicles (when compared to other species) indicate that we evolved when there was a lot of sexual competition and us gals had multiple sex partners. But on the other hand, the presence of oxytocin and arginine vasopressin receptors in the brain, both considered to be hormones that biologically promote monogamy, points to the fact that we seek to have one sexual partner at a time. A third major factor to consider is the presence of testosterone, which actually inhibits the receptor for oxytocin. Men have five to ten times more testosterone than women, and it drives them to seek more sexual partners. So what can we surmise from this multifaceted mess? "We have socially monogamous brains but sexually promiscuous genitals . . . Adding testosterone to the mix is like having a wild card in poker—anything can happen," says Paul J. Zak for *Psychology Today*.[78]

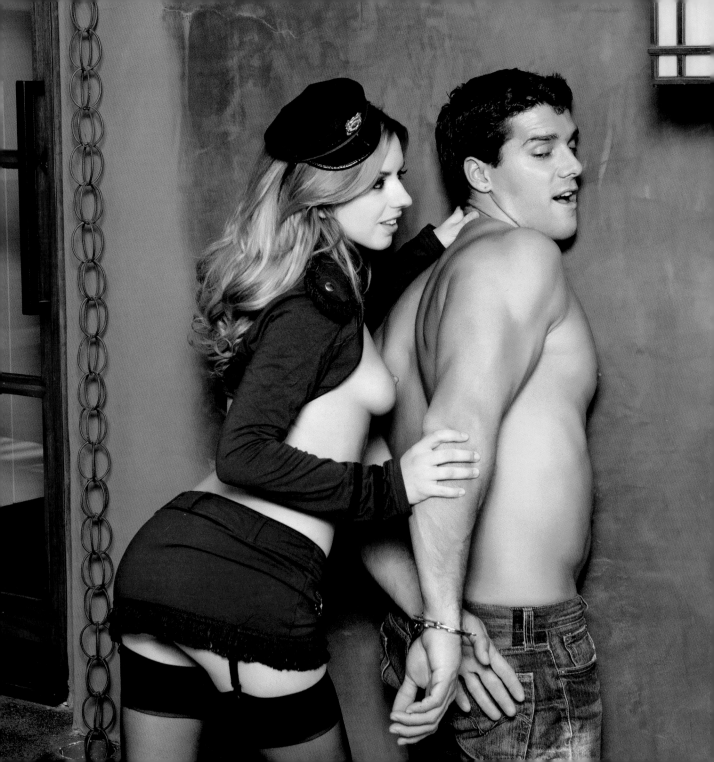

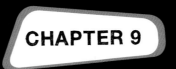

CHAPTER 9

DISORDERLY CONDUCT: DIFFICULT PROBLEMS THAT CAN POP UP

His dick is subject to a variety of disorders, both physical and psychosomatic, from ejaculation and erection difficulties to pains in the penis and sexually transmitted infections. In this chapter, we'll discuss some of the problems that can pop up and tell you how to successfully sexually navigate your way through them for a healthier Mr. Happy.

ERECTILE DYSFUNCTION

When His Erection Malfunctions

Erectile dysfunction (ED) is basically a fancy way of saying that he can't get it up. A temporary mechanical failure can happen to any guy–particularly in the case of whiskey dick, a condition resulting from consuming too much alcohol. Other times, the malfunction doesn't have as ready an explanation. Says fortysomething Colt, "ED happens to every guy over the age of twenty-five from time to time. I just ignore it and look forward to the next time." However, some men have erection problems more frequently and for more serious reasons, which can wreak havoc on their sex lives and their confidence.

The causes of ED fall into two broad categories: physical and psychological. How can you tell the difference? Well, does your guy get boners while he sleeps? If he is still constructing morning wood, his ED is all in his head. However, if his prick is floppy morning, noon, and night, he may have a physical condition that is blocking that all-important blood flow to his boner.

Physical Problems That Can Cause a Droopy Pee-pee

Diabetes, high blood pressure, obesity, vascular disease, surgery, side effects from smoking, drinking, drugs (prescribed or otherwise), and a host of other physical causes can disrupt an erection. (See chapter ten for more information on the relationship between his heart health and his hard-on.) Some of these problems are easily solved, such as taking medications to lower high blood pressure. But other problems may be more complex, such as in some cases of diabetes. Diabetes can damage the blood vessels and nerves that control erections.[81] Says sixtysomething Thomas, "I have diabetes, which causes ED. I've been unable to resolve it. So instead I induce orgasms in my partner with mouth and fingers and other preparations, like long warm-oil backrubs, candles, and champagne before and after."

Psychological Problems That Can Cause a Misbehaving Hard-on

Relationship stress such as cheating partners, financial troubles, or frequent arguing over who gets to wake up at 3 a.m. to change poopy diapers can all impede a boner. He may also have hang-ups left over from his religious upbringing (no one wants to go to hell for ejaculating), or from sexual abuse that occurred in his childhood.

The most common psychological problem is performance anxiety. This is a temporary manifestation of ED that results when a guy psychs himself out before the big (bedroom) game. If, for example, the first time he tries to please you in the sack his penis fails him, subsequent attempts may be foiled by his belief that he won't be able to get it up . . . ever again. Performance anxiety is the easiest issue to address, because all it takes is a little patience and encouragement to get him back into tip-top fucking condition. Says Jay, a fiftysomething technician, "ED happened to me only once. Funny thing is, I think it was because she was so excited to finally get to be with me and she kept telling me so, which made me feel pressured. She didn't get too upset with me when my erection failed, so everything ended up fine and the next morning we got to it."

> The most common psychological problem is performance anxiety. This is a temporary manifestation of ED that results when a guy psychs himself out before the big (bedroom) game.

Tips for Expertly Handling a Dysfunctional Erection

❶ **Don't blame yourself!** You might feel like you are somehow failing your man because you are unable to help him achieve an erection. Unless he lost his responsiveness after you had a threesome with his brother and best friend behind his back, the problem has nothing to do with you. Avoid the desire to ask him what you did wrong, and try not to overanalyze or pick apart the situation. It's best to let it slide, so he isn't stressed out about his erection the next time he has a chance to play (which can have a terrible snowball effect).

Men who aren't overly eager to stick it in you are often more patient and giving lovers. This is a great opportunity to employ tongue, fingers, and toys to achieve amazing and long-lasting pleasure.

2 Be compassionate. Men put a lot of stock in their ability to perform sexually. So whatever you do, don't poke fun at his suffering; this will only exacerbate the problem.

3 Think outside the cock. Sometimes the best sex is had without the usual penis-plunging-into-vagina action. Men who aren't overly eager to stick it in you are often more patient and giving lovers. This is a great opportunity to employ tongue, fingers, and toys to achieve amazing and long-lasting pleasure. You may find that you'll enjoy more and better orgasms.

4 Treasure his pleasure map. Your man can be sexually stimulated even with a slumbering penis. Massages, nibbling, tickling, and teasing him all over can bring him great pleasure. And who knows, thanks to the lack of performance pressure, he may even surprise you both by rising to the occasion!

5 Consult an M.D. If the problem is physical, your man should consult his doctor to see if the underlying health issue can be resolved. Sometimes, all it takes is quitting smoking or beginning an exercise routine and eating more vegetables to get his dick back in working order. If the problem is disease related, a physician may be able to assist by prescribing any of the ED medications available on the market today.

6 Consult a Ph.D. If the issue is psychological, usually patience, kindness, and time will work wonders to solve his mental hang-ups. But if he needs more help, your man should consult a licensed sex therapist who can work with him to uncover any underlying issues that are undermining what's in his underpants.

DELAYED EJACULATION

When the Train Won't Let Him Get Off

Delayed ejaculation refers to when a man requires extra-long lovin' to ejaculate (thirty minutes or more). It can also describe a condition in which he can't ejaculate at all, no matter how much stimulation he receives. Delayed ejaculation is only a problem if it negatively interferes with your sex life. Sometimes, the issue can be permanent, while other times it's only temporary, and, like ED, it can be caused by either physical or psychological issues. Lawrence, a twenty-nine-year-old playwright, says, "I suffered from delayed ejaculation. Often, I would stay hard for a very long time without being able to come. This was [based on] a psychological fear of getting a girl pregnant. I have overcome it somewhat, but it still takes me a while."

Antidepressants and high blood pressure medications, as well as marijuana and alcohol abuse, can cause delayed ejaculation. Other physical causes include birth defects, spinal cord injury, surgery, prostate or urinary tract infections, and diabetes. Delayed ejaculation should not be confused with retrograde ejaculation, which is when your guy orgasms but doesn't spurt. In cases of retrograde ejaculation, his semen has gone the wrong way down the sperm highway and exited into his bladder.

Tips for Handling Your "Love You Long Time" Lover

❶ **Enjoy it.** If your guy's delayed ejaculation is not a symptom of a larger health concern, take advantage of his endurance sex. You may find that his sexual response cycle is more in line with your own and that he'll last long enough to allow you to achieve your sought-after orgasm. (Or if you're even luckier—multiple orgasms!)

2 **Warm him up.** If your pussy gets tired after, say, more than 100 thrusts, get him started long before penetration. Have him masturbate for you, give him a warm-up blow job, or use a sex toy (such as a masturbation sleeve) on him to get things heated up. When he's obviously getting closer to ejaculation, you can send in your home-run hitter.

3 **Lay off the booze and drugs.** If your guy is a heavy drinker or drug user, adopting a healthier lifestyle can bring him that much closer to being able to achieve his goals (including spurting like Old Faithful).

4 **See an M.D.** If you suspect his problem is related to prescription medications or an underlying health issue, see a doctor.

5 **See a Ph.D.** If your guy can't come due to debilitating psychological issues stemming from childhood sexual abuse, religious indoctrination, depression, or relationship stresses, he should see a sex therapist to overcome these hurdles.

PREMATURE EJACULATION

When His Hose Springs a Leak

Premature ejaculation (PE) describes the sexual situation in which your guy ejaculates sooner than he would like to. This becomes problematic when his hasty hard-on consistently makes it to the big-O finish line before you do. Any committed girl who has to rely solely on BOB (battery-operated boyfriend) to achieve all of her orgasms knows that PE can become a bit exasperating. Lucky for you and your little friend, the problem is usually an easy fix and you might be able to leave BOB in the drawer next time you do the mattress mambo.

Tips for Handling Your "Quick Draw McGraw"

❶ Play red light, green light. The easiest, most natural, and effective way to combat PE is known as the start-stop method.[82] First, your guy needs to rate his arousal on a scale of 1 to 10, 1 being getting a cavity filled and 10 being spurting cum all over your breasts. At a 3 or 4 he's feeling hard and horny, at a 7 or 8 he's thrusting with gusto, and at 9, he's only a few pumps away from shooting his spunk. During a sexual encounter, have your guy bring himself to about level 7, but before he pushes any further he must stop everything (red light!) until he relaxes back to a level 3 or 4, at which point he can rev his engines back up (green light!). Have him repeat this sequence three full times before allowing orgasm. The first few times he tries this method, it should be done alone with the aid of only Rosy Palms (or Palm à la Handerson). When he's mastered it with those two handy assistants, the two of you can practice together. Start by using your hands and lube, and eventually try it inside the overwhelmingly arousing confines of your body. Be patient and allow him plenty of practice. Over time, your guy will learn how to extend his performance and ejaculate at will—a boon for the both of you!

❷ Foreplay! It's common for women to take longer to achieve orgasm than men. For a woman who is dating a man with a much shorter arousal cycle than her own, foreplay is the best way to obtain mutual satisfaction. Make it a household rule that you always come first and encourage your three-pump chump to bring you to your big O before he gets invited inside to play. Most women find satisfaction in a little (or a lotta) oral or finger play before penetration. To add more excitement, reveal your secret dildo and let him do the dirty work while you lie back and enjoy the sensations. Only when he's successfully driven you over the crest of orgasm hill can he climb on for his own ride.

 Make it a household rule that you always come first and encourage your three-pump chump to bring you to your big O before he gets invited inside to play.

Because sex is a human-to-human interaction that involves the exchange of a veritable cocktail of bodily fluids (more than you'd ever exchange by sharing a carton of milk), the risk of sexually transmitted infections should be taken seriously.

❸ **Extending creams.** There are a variety of desensitizing creams available at sex toy stores. These creams usually use benzocaine, which is a numbing agent (of the type you'd find in products that numb mouth sores, for example). The idea is to desensitize him to the pleasures of your pussy so that it will take him longer to come. Before you buy, do your research and read reviews by other users. Some creams have a bitter flavor, which means you won't be able to give him a blow job, while others are so strong that they'll have the unfortunate side effect of numbing you in the process (using a condom will help with this issue), and other creams just don't work at all.

❹ **Cock rings.** Wrap one of these little devices around the base of your man's prick to trap blood in his penis, allowing for bigger and longer-lasting erections. (For more info on how to use a cock ring, read chapter three.)

❺ **Priligy.** Drug manufacturers are jumping on the sexual dysfunction gravy train and trying to find a bona fide boner extender. Priligy is one of the newest in the line of defense against premature ejaculation. It's in the final stages of approval with the FDA, and is already prescribed in many European countries.[83] However, please note that drugs should always be a last resort in any sexual challenge. The best way to be a sexually functioning human being is to learn to work with your body.

SEXUALLY TRANSMITTED INFECTIONS

(Beware! Contagious!)

Because sex is a human-to-human interaction that involves the exchange of a veritable cocktail of bodily fluids (more than you'd ever exchange by sharing a carton of milk), the risk of sexually transmitted infections (STIs) should be taken seriously. Before toying with your boy toy, you'll want to find out if your partner is drug and disease free. (Sometimes, this isn't possible, especially if you are jumping into bed with that hotty you met in the produce section. It's not typical to discuss sexual histories while flirting over ripe fruit.) Ultimately, the best way to prevent STIs is to be in a committed monogamous relationship, but if that isn't preferable to you, use condoms every single time.

Chlamydia

Chlamydia shows its ugly face on the penis by way of inflammation of the urinary tract, causing painful peeing or a discharge of pus or mucus from the meatus. Symptoms usually occur within three weeks of exposure. Treatment for chlamydia is simple and consists of a short series of antibiotics. If untreated, your guy's nuts may swell up like balloons, and he could develop a painful reactive arthritis called Reiter syndrome, which is a real pain in the penis and can cause lesions, incontinence, and other unsavory issues.[84]

Gonorrhea

Gonorrhea is chlamydia's ugly sister and shows up in the form of a white or yellowish discharge from the penis accompanied by a painful burning sensation while urinating. Your guy can also get the gunk in his rectum, causing an itching butthole and painful poops. Symptoms usually occur within ten days of exposure. Usually, gonorrhea is treated at the same time as chlamydia with a simple series of antibiotics.[85]

Human Papillomavirus

Human papillomavirus, or HPV, is one of the most common STIs, and it comes in at least sixty different viral flavors. The Center for Disease Control (CDC) reports that at least 50 percent of sexually active people will get some form of HPV in their lives. Some varieties of HPV can cause penile cancer, which is rare. Unfortunately, it isn't easy to spot a prick with HPV, because it's uncommon for a man to manifest any symptoms. Only a few strains of the virus show up as occasional outbreaks of genital warts. Moreover, women are susceptible to developing cervical cancer as a result of the virus.

The CDC recommends that men aged twenty-six or younger receive the Gardasil vaccine, which will protect them from most strains of HPV that cause genital warts. Condoms may lower the risk of HPV, but because the virus is transmitted from skin-to-skin contact, condoms won't cover the entire affected area (such as the pubic region and testicles), and aren't 100 percent effective.[86]

Genital Herpes

Herpes infect about 16 percent of Americans between fourteen and forty-nine years old, including one out of nine men. It's more likely for a man to give a woman this unwanted gift than the other way around. Herpes show up as blistering sores on the genitals that last from several days to several weeks, and will pop up randomly as long as a person is carrying the virus (which typically lasts a lifetime). Between outbreaks, it will appear to be all systems normal. However, these tricky buggers can be transmitted even when there are no sores. It's best to use condoms at all times, which can reduce the risk of sharing this fun little virus. The use of antiviral medications can help prevent outbreaks, and some people with frequent outbreaks (six or more times per year) can be put on daily suppressive therapy (a daily dose of antiviral meds such as Valtrex) to prevent sores from rearing their icky lil' heads.[87]

Syphilis

Syphilis has plagued civilization since the sixteenth century. Before the days of penicillin, it could not be treated and caused the suffering and death of many. Perhaps this is why the Italian physician Girolamo Fracastoro saw fit to write an epic poem, which he titled "Syphilis" (1530), to describe the effects of the disease (which he blamed on the French) and to give it a namesake. "What were the varied accidents of matter, what the seeds which brought on an unaccustomed disease through long centuries seen by no one, which in our time raged through all Europe, parts of Asia and through the cities of Africa? It burst into Italy with the unhappy French wars and took its name from that people."[88]

Today, the syphilis bacteria still infects people (in the United States, 36,000 cases were reported in 2006), but is usually discovered and treated early with a dose of antibiotics. There are four stages of this nasty disease. In the first stage, a single, small chancre sore develops on the genitals. In the second stage, the chancre will disappear and be replaced by a rash of rough red spots on the hands and feet, sometimes accompanied by flu-like symptoms, weight loss, and hair loss. In the third stage, the rash and symptoms will disappear and the syphilis will stay latent in the body for up to twenty years before attacking the organs, including the brain, liver, eyes, bones, and more. The last stage can cause paralysis, numbness, dementia, blindness, and death. Prevent this from happening to you (and your lovers) by using condoms and regularly getting tested for syphilis along with other STIs.[89]

Crabs (Pubic Lice)

Crabs are not transmitted from swimming in dirty ocean water (contrary to what your friends might have told you in junior high). These unpleasant little parasites are sexually transmitted. Unlike many other STIs, the symptoms are obvious throughout the infection. They cause itching and, if looked at closely, you can see them with the naked eye. Crabs cozy up in the coarse pubic hair in the form of eggs, which eventually hatch and grow into adults. Contrary to urban legend, you cannot contract crabs from toilet seats, because they can't survive outside the moist, warm environment of the human body. Every so often, crabs will infest underarm hair, eyelashes, beards, and eyebrows. To get rid of these disgusting creatures, try over-the-counter lice-killing lotions. If this doesn't work, visit your doctor for a prescription-strength solution.[90]

> Contrary to urban legend, you cannot contract crabs from toilet seats, because they can't survive outside the moist, warm environment of the human body.

Priapism (named after Priapus, the Greek god of fertility) is a painful erection that develops for nonsexual reasons and won't go away. Physiologically, blood becomes trapped in the penis. Priapism is often caused by ED medications gone haywire.

HIV/AIDS

HIV/AIDS is the most pernicious STI of our time. HIV is a human immunodeficiency virus that leads to AIDS (acquired immunodeficiency syndrome). The first known case of the infection was detected in a blood sample taken from a man in the Democratic Republic of the Congo in 1959. Researchers believe the virus originated in chimpanzees in West Africa and was introduced to human hunters who came in contact with their blood. The disease became a full blown epidemic in the United States in the 1980s.

HIV attacks the immune system and can cause rapid deterioration in health by making sufferers more susceptible to diseases such as pneumonia and cancers that cause death. HIV/AIDS is transmitted by direct exposure to blood and semen and is thus most commonly transmitted via unprotected sex and intravenous drug use with shared needles. Unlike STIs that are transmitted from skin-to-skin contact, the virus is highly preventable during sex by using condoms. More than twenty years of medical research and progress have produced drugs that actively and effectively suppress the virus and allow people to live fairly normal lives. Also, a drug cocktail known as antiretroviral therapy, or ART, has been shown to decrease the risk of HIV transmission.[91],[92] However, this STI stands alone as reason enough to always practice safer sex.

PENIS-SPECIFIC PROBLEMS

(Icky, but Not Contagious!)

Since these odd little issues can surface on any penis, it's a good idea to learn how to recognize them and know what to do about them.

Peyronie's Disease

If you notice your man's penis bending at an extreme angle and sex has become painful for him, he may have Peyronie's disease (named after the eighteenth century French surgeon, François de la Peyronie, who first documented the disease). The condition is caused by a series of microfractures or traumas (e.g., getting hit in the crotch with a baseball, or bending his penis in a sloppy attempt to copulate) that lead to calcification, scarring, and deformation of the penis. In some cases, the issue will resolve itself over time. Other cases may be treated with prescribed oral medicines and injections, and severe cases may require surgery.[93]

Priapism

Priapism (named after Priapus, the Greek god of fertility) is a painful erection that develops for nonsexual reasons and won't go away. Physiologically, blood becomes trapped in the penis. Priapism is often caused by ED medications gone haywire (thus, the classic warning: If you take Viagra and you experience an erection that lasts four or more hours, you should seek medical attention). Other causes include sickle-cell anemia, genital trauma, black widow spider bites, and cocaine and marijuana use. To treat the problem, apply ice packs to his genitals. If this doesn't make the erection subside, your guy will have to head to the emergency room, where they may have to aspirate his penis by inserting a needle and draining blood from his boner. In some extreme cases, his penis may be injected with a drug that causes his veins to narrow and reduce blood flow, or surgical intervention may be required.[94]

Balanitis

Balanitis (named after the Greek word *balanos* meaning "acorn") is an inflammation of the skin of his glans and is more common among uncircumcised males with poor hygiene. The condition can be brought about by a buildup of smegma under the foreskin, which, in turn, causes a stinky, itchy, inflamed rash. Balanitis can also be caused by diabetes, obesity, penile cancer, an allergy to soaps, spermicides or other products, a yeast infection, or it can be the result of an STI. If your man develops this condition, he should seek medical attention immediately so that the underlying cause can be determined and he can be treated appropriately by a physician.[95,96]

While we like to think that sex is always fun and carefree, it's good to remember that sometimes problems can pop up. The best way to equip yourself to handle these sticky or icky situations is to educate yourself, take precautions, and act when necessary.

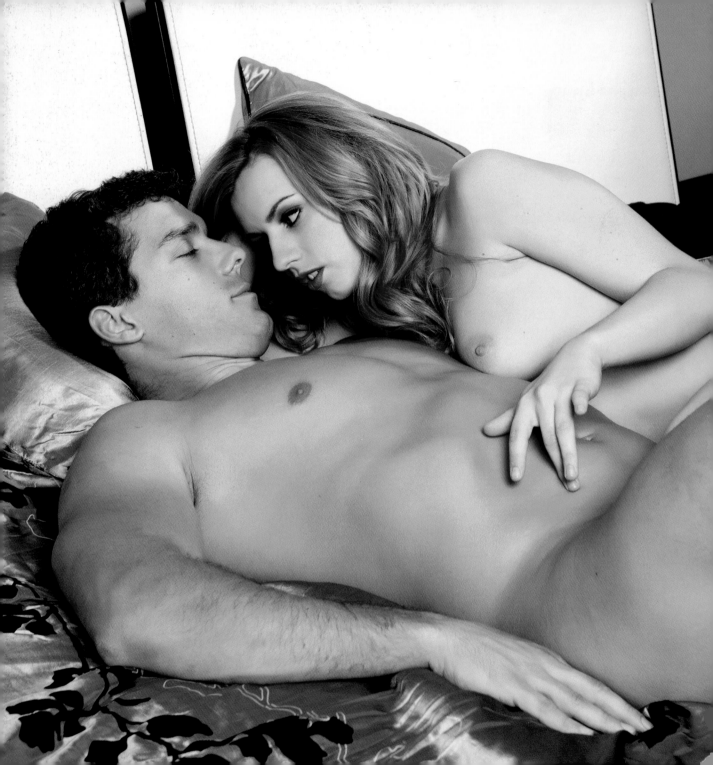

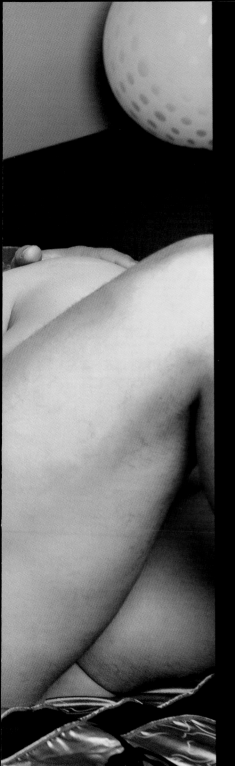

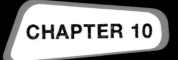
A HAPPY, HEALTHY PENIS: PROTECTING YOUR (AND HIS) FAVORITE PLAYTHING FOR A LIFETIME

Just as he takes extra-special care of his sports car, motorcycle, or boat, your guy should take care of his penis as if it were a valuable possession. After all, a sexy sex life is an important component to a happy life, and the health of his cock is linked to his overall health. Let's talk about the best ways to take care of your (and his) favorite plaything for life.

Exercise thirty to sixty minutes per day . . . and yes, a little vigorous sex counts toward his total! This will help him keep his weight down, keep his heart healthy, and keep his erections going strong.

KEGEL EXERCISES: WHAT ARE THEY GOOD FOR?

Kegel exercises were initially developed by the gynecologist Dr. Arnold Kegel (1894-1981) to help treat women who developed urinary incontinence after childbirth. However, the technique isn't only beneficial to women. It's also been found to help men keep their prostates healthy, avoid incontinence, increase sexual pleasure, and even treat premature ejaculation. Even with all these benefits, only 40 percent of the men we surveyed say they do their Kegels, and of these men, a third do them only occasionally, when they think about it. Eighteen percent of men admitted they don't even know what Kegels are!

Kegel exercises are performed by squeezing the pubococcygeus (PC) muscle of the pelvic floor. The PC muscle cradles the pelvic area in both men and women, running from the pubic bone to the tailbone. When he squeezes his PC muscle, he may feel a lift to his testicles and a tightening of the anal sphincter muscle.[97] Performed daily, Kegels will improve the long-term health of his private parts. For information on how to do this exercise, read on.

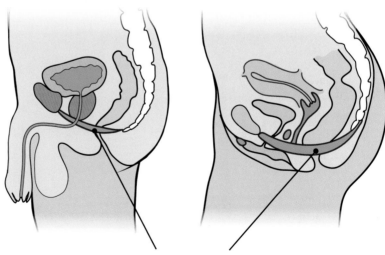

PC muscles in a man and woman

HIS HEART AND HIS COCK—A LOVE AFFAIR

A man's erection can be directly related to the health of his heart. If your man has difficulty getting or maintaining boners, it may be the first sign that his heart isn't working quite right. Both his penis and his heart rely on healthy arteries to keep the blood flowing. The smaller arteries in his penis will likely start showing signs of clogging sooner than the larger arteries in his heart. Although a sad erection could indicate a problem with his figurative heart (say he's feeling blue over a fight you had with each other and just isn't in the mood), it can also represent a more literal warning sign of developing health problems such as cardiovascular disease. Other warning signs that the problem could be with his ticker (and not just his prick) include if he has diabetes, if he is younger than fifty and experiencing ED, if he is overweight, smokes, has high blood pressure, is depressed, or has a family history of heart disease. If any of these problems sound familiar, encourage your guy to see his doctor for an evaluation.[99]

Tips for Keeping His Boner (and Heart) Healthy

❶ **Quit smoking.** There are some 4,800 chemicals in tobacco smoke, and many are damaging to the heart and blood vessels. Nicotine narrows his blood vessels and increases heart rate and blood pressure. Carbon monoxide saps the blood of oxygen, and his heart has to work even harder to oxygenate the blood. Because his hard-on requires healthy blood flow, the narrowing blood vessels and easily fatigued heart mean fewer and weaker erections. Not to mention, who wants to kiss a guy with smoker's breath? Motivate your man to put out his cigarette, for good, with the promise of a healthier sex life.

❷ **Exercise** thirty to sixty minutes per day . . . and yes, a little vigorous sex counts toward his total! This will help him keep his weight down, keep his heart healthy, and keep his erections going strong. Men who exercise report a direct correlation between frequency of

SCIENTIFICALLY SPEAKING: WHAT IS PROSTATE CANCER?

Prostate cancer develops in the gland cells, which are responsible for producing prostate fluid, part of that creamy concoction known as semen. Most of the time prostate cancer grows slowly over a long period of time, although sometimes it grows rapidly. Prostate cancer is the second leading cause of cancer-related death in men (behind lung cancer) and affects about one in thirty-five men. It's more common in men over fifty years old, African Americans, and men who have a history of prostate cancer in their family. Early prostate cancer usually does not come with symptoms. A man aged fifty and over (or forty and over if he has a history of prostate cancer in his family) should talk to his physician to find out whether he should be screened for prostate cancer. Scientists still don't know exactly what causes prostate cancer; however, the American Cancer Society suggests that a healthy diet that includes lots of fruits and vegetables, and limits red meat and processed foods, can help decrease his risk of developing the disease.[109]

exercise and frequency of sex. This could be a side effect of their chiseled abs and improved confidence, or a side effect of their extra healthy erections . . . or both!

3 **Eat right.** Encourage your guy to stop making trips to the drive thru and snack aisle where they serve fatty, salty, and sugary erection-preventing foodlike products. He should swap these out for a diet full of fruits, vegetables, legumes, lean proteins, and plenty of water. Diet not only affects heart health, but it also affects his mood. A good diet means a good mood, which means more excitement when it comes to getting your clothes off and having his way with you.

4 **Alcohol in moderation.** Men can drink up to two alcoholic beverages per day (red wine is the best) for heart health. The relaxing effects of the alcohol can also help inspire a bit of exciting bedroom action. However, if he ups the ante to three or more servings of alcohol, he not only puts his heart at risk, but he puts himself at risk of getting whiskey dick and not being able to perform in the sack.

5 **Checkups.** Your man should see his doctor at least once a year. Be sure he is checked for both blood pressure and cholesterol and is tested for sexually transmitted infections (especially if he has more than one sex partner). Remember, an ounce of prevention leads to hours of amazing sex. A good bill of health will encourage him to stay on track, and make for even better lovemaking.[103]

EJACULATION IS GOOD FOR HIM

In 1892, Dr. John Harvey Kellogg wrote, " . . . when seminal losses occur more frequently than once a month, they will certainly ultimate in great injury, even though immediate ill effects are not noticed." He attributed conditions such as enlarged prostates, urinary infections, heart disease, epilepsy . . . pretty much anything that can go wrong with his health . . . to semen loss and argued that men should lose their semen no more than once per month, and less would be better.[104]

Today's scientists argue that the opposite is true. Ejaculation is good for him, and because it doesn't carry the same risks of acquiring sexually transmitted infections, ejaculation via masturbation is even better.

In a 2004 study carried out by the National Cancer Institute, 342 men were evaluated over the course of eight years, during which time frequency of ejaculation was compared with the development of prostate cancer. The study found that "high ejaculation frequency was related to *decreased* risk of total prostate cancer." Men who masturbated twenty-one or more times per month fared better than those who ejaculated four to seven times per month.[105]

This study is backed up by another conducted in 2003 by Graham Giles of the Cancer Council Australia. The researchers found that men who ejaculated five times or more per week in their twenties were one-third less likely to develop prostate cancer later.[106] In an interview with *New Scientist*, Giles attributed his findings to what he calls the "prostatic stagnation hypothesis," which basically proposes that men who ejaculate frequently cleanse their prostates and help prevent the buildup of carcinogens.[107] Perhaps there is a shadow of truth, then, behind the urban myth DSB (deadly sperm backup). DSB is the male equivalent of PMS and is said to occur when a man isn't getting laid enough, which causes moodiness and sometimes death.[108] Next time your man is whining over the remote and cracking open your chocolate almond fudge ice cream, lovingly remind him that it may be time for him to "crack one off" instead.

Next time your man is whining over the remote and cracking open your chocolate almond fudge ice cream, lovingly remind him that it may be time for him to "crack one off" instead.

LAB WORK: KEGELS, NOW!

Purpose:
To determine whether practicing Kegel exercises improves the quality of sex and orgasms for either or both of you

What you'll need:
His penis, lab notebook, pencil, white lab coat (lingerie optional), a little patience, and a bossy attitude

The method:

1 While having sex one evening, slow the process down and squeeze his penis with your pelvic muscles. Ask him to return the favor. When you feel him expand inside of you, tell him how good it feels and suggest that you should both start practicing your Kegels.

2 First, he'll need to learn how to do Kegel exercises, especially if this is the first time he's tried them. To find the PC muscle, he should stop the flow of urine while he's peeing. If he can, he's successfully found his PC muscle.

3 Now he can practice his Kegels outside of the bathroom. To properly exercise this muscle, he needs to follow these steps: squeeze, hold, release, rest, and repeat. First squeeze and draw the muscle up and in

around his anus and urethra. Strongly hold this contraction for as long as he can (one to ten seconds). Now release and rest for ten seconds. Repeat the sequence up to twelve times. After he's accomplished the long hold, he can try five to ten fast contractions. He should *not* hold his breath or contract his abs, butt, or thighs while doing these exercises—that would be cheating![98]

4 It would be easy for him to neglect to do his exercises, but not with you, his sexy scientist, there to keep tabs. So put him on a reminder system. Perhaps you can lean over and whisper "Kegels, now!" while you are seated in a crowded theater or at dinner with the in-laws. Or call (or text) him while he's at the office, simply say "Kegels, now!" and hang up. You'll have him under your erotic command and no one will be the wiser. His exercises should be done daily.

5 He should also practice performing a few contractions during intercourse. This will cause his penis to swell inside you, and it will feel quite delightful.

6 It will take anywhere from three to six weeks for a marked

difference in the strength and endurance of his PC muscle to develop. Over time, he may be able to actually lift his testicles when he squeezes (he'll develop control over the cremaster muscle, which usually raises and lowers his scrotum involuntarily, as it does when his nuts are cold and need to be warmed up close to his body). Keep tabs on his progress in your lab notebook and note any changes in the following areas:

- Time it takes for him to ejaculate
- Improvements in your orgasmic experience
- Improvements in his orgasmic experience
- Any other notable changes

7 For even better results, practice *your* Kegels (using the same techniques) right along with him. Have fun!

The conclusion:
You'll find that bringing awareness to your sexual health will add a new dimension of pleasure to your sex games. Encouraging each other to develop in positive ways not only enhances the well-being of your bodies, but also of your relationship.

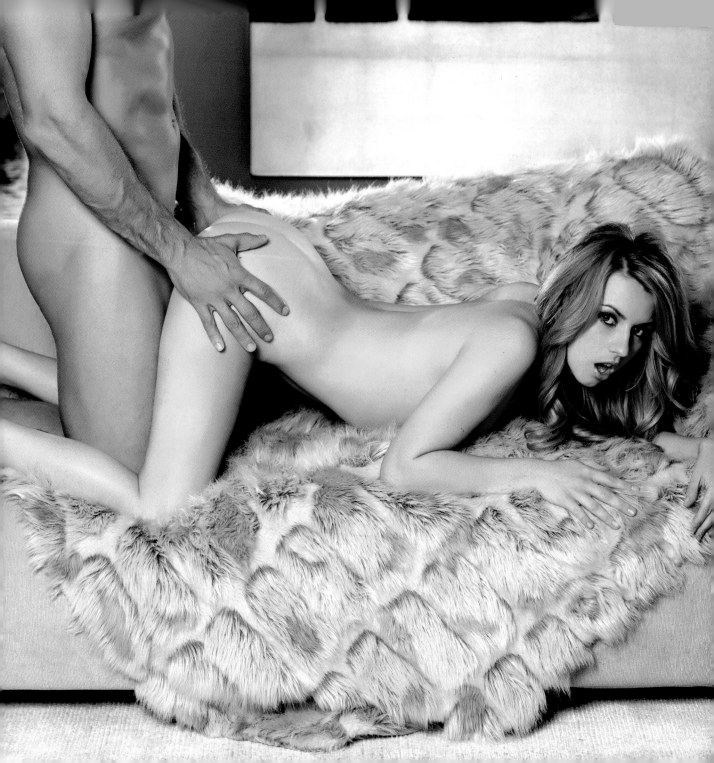

Tips on Healthy Ejaculation

How frequently a man can ejaculate depends on multiple factors, including his overall health, his age, and his unique sex drive. Here are some ways you can make sure he's keeping his prostate clear and ready for takeoff:

❶ **Learn how to give a prostate massage.** If what scientists are saying is true, giving prostate massages can keep the fluids flowing and help prevent bad stuff from backing up in his pipes. (Read chapter four for more information on how to give a prostate massage.)

❷ **Participate in the fun.** With his sexy scientist around, your man doesn't have to always go it alone. Masturbate with him and add a little excitement to your sexual repertoire. Pick out a porn movie together, or order a set of his and hers sex toys and enjoy the fun of mutual masturbation. You can either masturbate each other, or enjoy your own private voyeur/exhibitionist game.

❸ **Sex is good for you.** Make it a goal to increase the number of times you and your partner have sex. If you partner up once a month, try going for it once per week. If you have a once-weekly ritual, up the ante to three or four times per week. If you are already going at it like bunnies, kudos to you! You'll find that the more sex you have, the more you'll both want.

A happy penis brings with it the benefits of better overall health and a more satisfying sex life. Keep your plaything in top condition by practicing Kegels, observing a healthy and active lifestyle, and enjoying frequent sex, and you'll both reap great rewards in and out of the bedroom.

SCIENTIFICALLY SPEAKING— SEXY VITAMINS

Certain nutrients and vitamins are key to keeping his sexual machinery well oiled. Make sure he's getting enough of these to keep him in tip-top condition (many of these vitamins contribute to his general, overall health, as well):

1. **Zinc** has a wide range of functions in the body, including being an important component of semen and sperm (there is approximately 100 times as much zinc in semen as there is in the blood). Because of this, men require more zinc than women, and the more times he blows his load, the more zinc he'll need. The recommended daily amount of zinc for grown men is around 9.5 mg (but be careful, too much zinc can be toxic).[100]

2. **Vitamin E** plays an important role in sperm production, as well as the production of key sex hormones and enzymes.

3. **Ginkgo biloba** relaxes artery walls, thus increasing blood circulation in his body and blood flow to his boner.

4. **L-arginine** also increases blood flow to the nether regions and can help provide a longer-lasting, harder erection.[101]

5. **Vitamin B complex** will improve energy and circulation (B1 and B3), aid in the production of sex hormones (B3), and has been associated with preventing erectile dysfunction (B12).

6. **Vitamin C** is key in promoting the healthy lining of arteries, which provides for more and healthier hard-ons.[102]

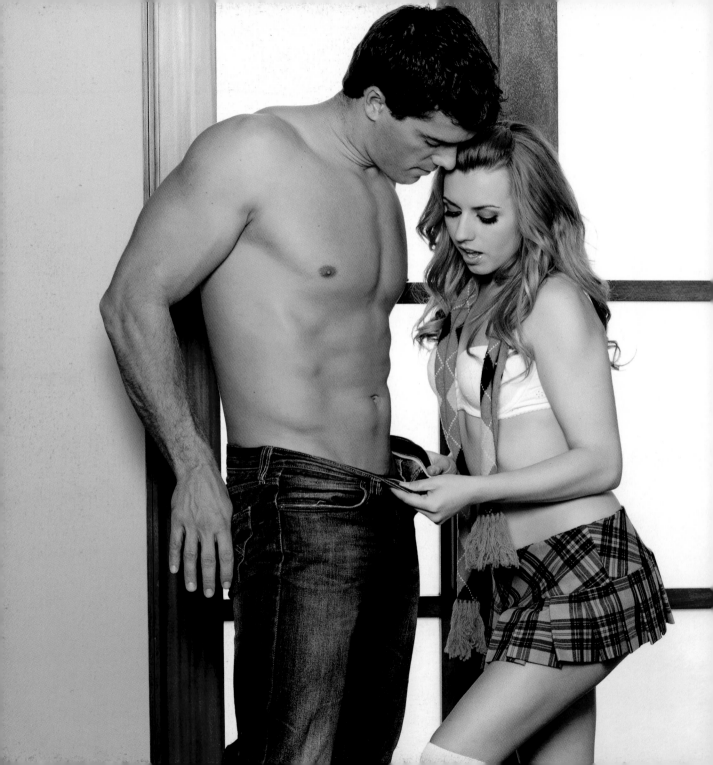

ENDNOTES

1   Masters, William H., and Virginia E. Johnson. *Human Sexual Response*. Toronto: Bantam, 1981. Print, p. 178.

2   Masters, William H., and Virginia E. Johnson, pp. 179–80.

3   Greenberg, Jerrold S., Clint E. Bruess, and Sarah C. Conklin. *Exploring the Dimensions of Human Sexuality*. Sudbury, Mass.: Jones and Bartlett, 2007. Print, p. 365.

4   Bering, Jesse. "Secrets of the Phallus: Why Is the Penis Shaped Like That?" *Scientific American*. 27 Apr. 2009. Web, 14 June 2010. http://www.scientificamerican.com/article.cfm?id=secrets-of-the-phallus.

5   Gallup, Jr., Gordon G., and Rebecca L. Burch. "Semen Displacement as a Sperm Competition Strategy in Humans." *Evolutionary Psychology* 2 (2004): 12–23. Web. http://www.epjournal.net/filestore/ep021223.pdf.

6   Strong, Bryan. *Human Sexuality: Diversity in Contemporary America*. New York: McGraw Hill, 2008. Print, p. 106.

7   Adams, Cecil. "The Straight Dope: What Is the Plural of 'penis'?" *The Straight Dope—Fighting Ignorance Since 1973*. 13 Jan. 2004. Web, 14 June 2010. http://www.straightdope.com/columns/read/2139/what-is-the-plural-of-penis.

8   "Frenulum | Define Frenulum at Dictionary.com." *Dictionary.com, Find the Meanings and Definitions of Words at Dictionary.com*. 2010. Web, 14 June 2010. http://dictionary.reference.com/browse/frenulum.

9   "Frenulum Clitoridis: Definition with Frenulum Clitoridis Pictures and Photos." *Lexicus—Word Definitions for Puzzlers and Word Lovers*. 05 Mar. 2000. Web, 14 June 2010. http://www.lexic.us/definition-of/frenulum_clitoridis.

10   Cope, Jonathan. "Ouch!" *The Guardian, Guardian.co.uk*. 28 Feb. 2002. Web, 15 June 2010. http://www.guardian.co.uk/lifeandstyle/2002/feb/28/healthandwellbeing.health2.

11   Hammond, T. "A Preliminary Poll of Men Circumcised in Infancy or Childhood." *NOHARMM* Access Page. BJU International, Jan. 1999. Web, 14 June 2010. http://www.noharmm.org/bju.htm.

12   "Foreskin Sexual Function/Circumcision Sexual Dysfunction." *CIRP*. 9 Aug. 2008. Web, 14 June 2010. http://www.cirp.org/library/sex_function/.

13   Strong, Bryan, p. 107.

14   Strong, Bryan, p. 109.

15   Strong, Bryan, p. 110.

16   Dean, Dr. John. "Semen and Sperm Quality." *NetDoctor.co.uk, The UK's Leading Independent Health Website*. 4 Apr. 2005. Web, 14 June 2010. http://www.netdoctor.co.uk/menshealth/facts/semenandsperm.htm.

17   Edell, Dr. Dean. "Why Is My Semen Watery?" *HealthCentral.com, Trusted, Reliable and Up-to-Date Health Information*. 27 Aug. 2001. Web, 14 June 2010. http://www.healthcentral.com/drdean/408/57960.html.

18   "Retrograde Ejaculation." *MayoClinic.com, Mayo Clinic Medical Information and Tools for Healthy Living*. 25 Mar. 2009. Web, 14 June 2010. http://www.mayoclinic.com/health/retrograde-ejaculation/ds00913.

19   Zimmer, Donald. "FAQ on Semen." *AskMen.com—Men's Online Magazine*. 28 Mar. 2007. Web, 14 June 2010. http://www.askmen.com/dating/dzimmer_100/117_love_answers.html.

20   Masters, William H., and Virginia E. Johnson, p. 212.

21   Sweet, Adam. "Disgusting World Records." *www.drinky.org.uk
     –The Site for the Debauched Intellectual.* Web, 14 June 2010.
     http://www.drinky.org.uk/stuff/disgusting.html.

22   Herbenick, Dr. Debby. "Semen in the Eye: Is It Dangerous? What
     Should I Do If I Get Sperm in My Eye? | My Sex Professor: Sexuality
     Education." *My Sex Professor: Sexuality Education from Sex Educator
     Dr. Debby Herbenick.* 15 Apr. 2009. Web, 14 June 2010. http://www.
     mysexprofessor.com/how-to-have-sex/semen-in-the
     -eye-is-it-dangerous-what-should-i-do/.

23   Werthman, Dr. Philip. "Center for Male Reproduction–
     Frequently Asked Questions." *Center for Male Reproduction
     & Vasectomy Reversal–Welcome.* 2008. Web, 14 June 2010.
     http://www.malereproduction.com/05_faqs.html.

24   Gaur, DS, MS Talekar, and VP Pathak. "Alcohol Intake and Cigarette
     Smoking: Impact of Two Major Lifestyle Factors on Male Fertility."
     Indian Journal of Pathology and Microbiology 53.1 (2010): 35-40.
     PubMed.gov. Web. http://www.ncbi.nlm.nih.gov/pubmed/20090219.

25   Werthman, Dr. Philip.
     http://www.malereproduction.com/05_faqs.html.

26   Jurewicz, J., W. Hanke, M. Radwan, and JP Bonde. "Environmental
     Factors and Semen Quality." *International Journal of Occupational
     Medicine and Environmental Health* 22.4 (2009): 305-29.
     PubMed.gov. Web. http://www.ncbi.nlm.nih.gov/pubmed/20053623.

27   Sheynkin, Y., M. Jung, P. Yoo, D. Schulsinger, and E. Komaroff.
     "Increase in Scrotal Temperature in Laptop Computer Users." *Human
     Reproduction (Oxford, England)* 20.2 (2005): 452-55. *PubMed.gov.*
     Web. http://www.ncbi.nlm.nih.gov/pubmed/15591087.

28   "Vasectomy: What to Expect." *Familydoctor.org.* American
     Academy of Family Physicians, May 2009. Web, 14 June 2010.
     http://familydoctor.org/online/famdocen/home/men/
     reproductive/195.html.

29   "Hair Spa." *Hari's Hair & Beauty.* Web, 14 June 2010.
     http://www.harissalon.com/hair-spa.cfm.

30 "Wheat Protein Just as Good as Shiny Hair for Bull Semen."
    BellaSugar Australia. 28 Oct. 2009. Web, 14 June 2010.
    http://www.bellasugar.com.au/Wheat-protein-just-good-shiny
    -hair-bull-semen-5880819.

31 "WikiAnswers—Is Sperm Good for Your Skin?" *WikiAnswers—
    The Q&A Wiki*. 14 Mar. 2006. Web, 14 June 2010.
    http://wiki.answers.com/Q/Is_sperm_good_for_your_skin.

32 Deliva, Donna. "CUM VS MOISTURIZER—Vice Settles the Score!" *Vice*.
    Sept. 2003. Web, 14 June 2010. http://www.viceland.com/int/v10n8/
    htdocs/cum.php.

33 Gallup Jr., GG, RL Burch, and SM Platek. "Does Semen Have
    Antidepressant Properties?" *Archives of Sexual Behavior* 31.3 (2002):
    289–93. *PubMed.gov*. Web. http://www.ncbi.nlm.nih.gov/
    pubmed/12049024.

34 Skyler, Dr. Jenni. "What's in YOUR Semen??" *Buffsecret Blog*.
    4 Apr. 2010. Web, 14 June 2010. http://buffsecret.wordpress.com
    /2010/04/04/whats-in-your-semen/.

35 "Watch Funny Hand Job Video | Break.com." *Break.com*.
    7 Dec. 2006. Web, 14 June 2010. http://www.break.com/
    usercontent/2006/12/7/funny-hand job-192860.

36 Hex, Webmaster. "Tips and Tricks to Stimulate the Prostate."
    Buzzle Web Portal: Intelligent Life on the Web. Web, 14 June 2010.
    http://www.buzzle.com/articles/tips-and-tricks-to-stimulate-the-
    prostate.html.

37 Strong, Bryan, p. 111.

38 Adams, Cecil. "The Straight Dope: Why Do Men Have Nipples?"
    The Straight Dope—Fighting Ignorance Since 1973. 18 May 1979.
    Web, 14 June 2010. http://www.straightdope.com/columns/read/85/
    why-do-men-have-nipples.

39 "Functions of the Foreskin." *Circumcision Resource Center*.
    Web, 14 June 2010. http://www.circumcision.org/foreskin.htm.

40 "Define 'Prepuce.'" *WordNet—Princeton University*.
    Web, 14 June 2010. http://wordnet.princeton.edu/.

41   "Circumcision: Not a 'Snip,' but 15 Square Inches."
     NOHARMM Access Page. 06 Sept. 2005. Web, 14 June 2010.
     http://www.noharmm.org/snip.htm.

42   Masters, William H., and Virginia E. Johnson, p. 190.

43   Fleiss, Paul M., and Frederick M. Hodges. *What Your Doctor May
     Not Tell You about Circumcision*. New York: Warner Books, 2002.
     Print, p. 24.

44   "Smegma." *Wikipedia, the Free Encyclopedia*. Web, 14 June 2010.
     http://en.wikipedia.org/wiki/Smegma.

45   Payne, Ph.D., Kimberly, Lea Thaler, Tuuli Kukkonen, Serge Carrier,
     and Yitzchak Binik, Ph.D. "Sensation and Sexual Arousal in
     Circumcised and Uncircumcised Men." *Journal of Sexual
     Medicine* 4.3 (2007): 667-74. Wiley InterScience. Web.
     http://www3.interscience.wiley.com/journal/118496134/abstract.

46   "Muslim Circumcision Practices." *History of Circumcision*.
     Web, 15 June 2010. http://www.historyofcircumcision.net/index
     .php?option=com_content&task=view&id=27&Itemid=0.

47   "What Were the Original Motivations Behind Routine Infant
     Circumcision in the West?" *CIRP.org*. Web, 15 June 2010.
     http://www.cirp.org/pages/whycirc.html.

48   Strong, Bryan, p. 398.

49   "What Does Circumcision Cost?" *Pregnancy and Parenting—From the
     Labor of Love*. Web, 15 June 2010. http://www.thelaboroflove
     .com/articles/what-does-circumcision-cost/.

50   Perlstein, MD., David. "Circumcision: The Surgical Procedure;
     What Is the Chance of a Complication from a Circumcision."
     MedicineNet.com. 12 Oct. 2007. Web, 15 June 2010.
     http://www.medicinenet.com/circumcision_the_surgical_procedure/.

51   "Circumcision Policy Statement—Task Force on Circumcision."
     AAP Policy—Journal of the American Academy of Pediatrics.
     American Academy of Pediatrics, 1 Sept. 2005. Web, 15 June 2010.
     http://aappolicy.aappublications.org/cgi/content/abstract/
     pediatrics;103/3/686.

52   Francken AB, HB van de Wiel, MF van Driel, and WC Weijmar Schultz. "What Importance Do Women Attribute to the Size of the Penis?" *National Center for Biotechnology Information, U.S. National Library of Medicine.* Web, 28 Apr. 2010. http://www.ncbi.nlm.nih.gov/pubmed/12429149.

53   "All Sex Positions." *Your Guide for Sex Tips.* KuMo Web Communications Corporation. Web, 28 Apr. 2010. http://www.sexinfo101.com/sexualpositions.shtml.

54   Shah, J., and N. Christopher. "Can Shoe Size Predict Penile Length?" *BJU International* 90.6 (2002): 586-87. Print.

55   Johanson, Sue. "The Penis—Various Info." *Talk Sex with Sue Johanson.* Talk Sex Productions, Inc. Web, 28 Apr. 2010. http://www.talksexwithsue.com/penis.html. and

56   Nugteren HM, GT Balkema, AL Pascal, WC Schultz, JM Nijman, and MF van Driel. "Penile Enlargement: From Medication to Surgery." *National Center for Biotechnology Information, U.S. National Library of Medicine.* Web. 28 Apr. 2010. http://www.ncbi.nlm.nih.gov/pubmed/20169492.

57   Johanson, Sue. http://www.talksexwithsue.com/penis.html.

58   Rowanchilde, Raven. "Male Genital Modification: A Sexual Selection Interpretation." *Human Nature* 7.2 (1996): 189-215. *SpringerLink.* Web. 15 June 2010. http://www.springerlink.com/content/p21408658770u551/.

59   Morrison, Cheyenne. "History of Body Piercing." *Painful Pleasures, The Piercing Temple.* 1998. Web, 15 June 2010. http://www.painfulpleasures.com/piercing_history.htm.

60   Angel, Elayne. *The Piercing Bible: The Definitive Guide to Safe Body Piercing.* Berkeley, CA: Celestial Arts, 2009. Print, p. 161.

61   Angel, Elayne. p. 259.

62   Vatsyayana, and Richard Francis Burton. *The Kama Sutra of Vatsyayana.* Stilwell, KS: Digireads.com, 2005. Print, p. 102.

63   Paley, Maggie. *The Book of the Penis.* New York, NY: Grove, 2000. Print, p. 142

64 "Ancient Tattooed Mummies." *Tattoo Artist Directory and Tattoo Design Portfolios*. 2008. Web, 15 June 2010. http://ill-use.com/home/illmagazine-mainmenu-2/tattoo-articles-mainmenu-120/85-ancient-tattoo-mummies.html.

65 "Samoa Tattoos." *Samoan Sensation—THE Site about Samoa*. 21 Apr. 2000. Web, 14 June 2010. http://www.samoa.co.uk/tattoos.html.

66 *Phallus.is*. The Icelandic Phallological Museum. Web, 15 June 2010. http://www.phallus.is/.

67 Elmo the Penis. "Hello! My Name's Elmo—and I'm a Big Prick." *The International Phallological Society*. Web, 15 June 2010. http://humanpenis.org/elmo.html.

68 Akiteng, Yangki C. "Karamojong Long Penis—Tribal Penis Stretching [NOT TRUE!] by Yangki Christine Akiteng, The Real People's Love Doctor." *SearchWarp Writers' Community*. 08 Feb. 2009. Web, 15 June 2010. http://searchwarp.com/swa432487-1-Karamojong-Long-Penis-Ritualistic-Penis-Stretching-And-Enlargement-Techniques.htm.

69 "Does Penis Enlargement Work?" *Thunder's Place*. Web, 15 June 2010. http://www.thundersplace.com/wheres_the_proof.html.

70 Wanjek, Christopher. "Penis Enlargement Products Come Up Short | LiveScience." *LiveScience | Science, Technology, Health & Environmental News*. 20 Feb. 2007. Web, 15 June 2010. http://www.livescience.com/health/070220_bad_mad_column.html.

71 "AUA—Policy Statements—Penile Augmentation Surgery." *American Urological Association*. Oct. 2008. Web, 15 June 2010. http://www.auanet.org/content/guidelines-and-quality-care/policy-statements/p/penile-augmentation-surgery.cfm.

72 Hamann, Stephan, Rebecca A. Herman, Carla L. Nolan, and Kim Wallen. "Men and Women Differ in Amygdala Response to Visual Sexual Stimuli." *Nature Neuroscience* 7 (2004): 411–16. *Nature Neuroscience*. 7 Mar. 2004. Web, 15 June 2010. http://www.nature.com/neuro/journal/v7/n4/full/nn1208.html.

73 "Sexual Photographs: Surprise! Men Look at Faces, Women Focus on Sexual Acts." *Science Daily: News & Articles in Science, Health, Environment & Technology*. 12 Apr. 2007. Web, 14 June 2010. http://www.sciencedaily.com/releases/2007/04/070412160210.htm.

74   Gerardi, Ph.D., Maryrose. "What Effects Can Stress Have On My Sex Life?" *ABCNews.com—Breaking News, Politics, Online News, World News, Feature Stories, Celebrity Interviews and More.* ABC News, 6 Feb. 2008. Web, 15 June 2010. http://abcnews.go.com/Health/StressReacting/story?id=4675556.

75   Hirsch, M.D., Alan. "Various Aromas Found to Enhance Male Sexual Response." *The Smell & Taste Treatment & Research Foundation.* Web, 15 June 2010. http://www.smellandtaste.org/index.cfm?action=research.sexual.

76   Smith, Tom W. "American Sexual Behavior: Trends, Socio-Demographic Differences, and Risk Behavior." *General Social Survey* 2006. *Norc.org.* National Opinion Research Center University of Chicago. Web, 15 June 2010. http://www.norc.org/NR/rdonlyres/2663F09F-2E74-436E-AC81-6FFBF288E183/0/AmericanSexualBehavior2006.pdf. p. 54.

77   Gardner, Kasey-Dee. "News: Cheaters Among Us : Video : Discovery News." *Discovery News: Earth, Space, Tech, Animals, Dinosaurs, History.* 8 Feb. 2010. Web, 15 June 2010. http://news.discovery.com/videos/news-cheaters-among-us.html.

78   Zak, Paul J. "Why Men Cheat—The Trouble with Tiger." *Psychology Today.* 25 Apr. 2010. Web, 15 June 2010. http://www.psychologytoday.com/blog/the-moral-molecule/201004/why-men-cheat.

79   Bower, Bruce. "Grown Men Swap Bodies with Virtual Girl." *Science News.* 5 June 2010. Web, 15 June 2010. http://www.sciencenews.org/view/generic/id/59143/title/Grown_men_swap_bodies_with_virtual_girl.

80   "Benin Alert Over 'Penis Theft' Panic." *BBC News.* 27 Nov. 2001. Web, 15 June 2010. http://news.bbc.co.uk/2/hi/africa/1678996.stm.

81   Baird, John M. "Erectile Dysfunction (Impotence) and Diabetes: Causes & Treatments." WebMD—Better Information. Better Health. 1 Jan. 2007. Web, 15 June 2010. http://www.webmd.com/erectile-dysfunction/guide/ed-diabetes.

82   Skyler, Jenni. *The Intimacy Institute*.
     http://www.theintimacyinstitute.org/.

83   "Dapoxetine and FDA Approval for Premature Ejaculation."
     Premature Ejaculation Cure. Web, 15 June 2010.
     http://www.prematureejaculation.org/reviews/dapoxetine.html.

84   "Chlamydia–Symptoms, Treatment and Prevention."
     Consumer Health News, Information and Resources Updated Daily.
     The Health Central Network, Inc., 1 Apr. 2009. Web, 15 June 2010.
     http://www.healthscout.com/ency/68/316/main.html.

85   "Gonorrhea–Symptoms, Treatment and Prevention."
     Consumer Health News, Information and Resources Updated Daily.
     The Health Central Network, Inc., 1 Apr. 2009. Web, 15 June 2010.
     http://www.healthscout.com/ency/68/722/main.html.

86   "Genital HPV Infection–CDC Fact Sheet." *Centers for Disease Control
     and Prevention*. Department of Health and Human Services. Web, 15
     June 2010. http://www.cdc.gov/std/hpv/stdfact-hpv.htm.

87   "Genital Herpes–CDC Fact Sheet." *Centers for Disease Control and
     Prevention*. Department of Health and Human Services. Web, 15 June
     2010. http://www.cdc.gov/std/Herpes/STDFact-Herpes.htm.

88   Becker, Barbara J. "Plagues and People–Excerpts from 'Syphilis' by
     Girolamo Fracastoro." *Department of History, University of California,
     Irvine*. 2005. Web, 14 June 2010. https://www.uci.edu/clients/
     bjbecker/PlaguesandPeople/week4b.html.

89   "Syphilis–CDC Fact Sheet." *Centers for Disease Control and
     Prevention*. Department of Health and Human Services. Web, 15 June
     2010. http://www.cdc.gov/std/syphilis/STDFact-Syphilis.htm.

90   "Pubic 'Crab' Lice: Fact Sheet." *Centers for Disease Control and
     Prevention*. Department of Health and Human Services. Web, 15 June
     2010. http://www.cdc.gov/lice/pubic/factsheet.html.

91   "HIV/AIDS Basics | Questions and Answers | CDC HIV/AIDS." *Centers
     for Disease Control and Prevention*. Department of Health and
     Human Services. Web, 15 June 2010. http://www.cdc.gov/hiv/
     resources/qa/definitions.htm.

92   Steenhuysen, Julie. "Drug Cocktails Cut Couples' HIV Transmission Risk." *Reuters.com*. 26 May 2010. Web, 15 June 2010. http://www.reuters.com/article/idUSTRE64P6X520100526.

93   "Peyronie's Disease." *National Kidney and Urologic Diseases Information Clearinghouse*. Apr. 2009. Web, 15 June 2010. http://kidney.niddk.nih.gov/kudiseases/pubs/peyronie/index.htm.

94   "Priapism." *Cleveland Clinic*. 6 Feb. 2007. Web, 15 June 2010. http://my.clevelandclinic.org/disorders/priapism/hic_priapism.aspx.

95   "Disorders of the Penis." *Cleveland Clinic*. 10 Jan. 2007. Web, 15 June 2010. http://my.clevelandclinic.org/disorders/penile _disorders/hic_disorders_of_the_penis.aspx.

96   Leber, MD, Mark J., and Anuritha Tirumani, MD. "Balanitis: eMedicine Emergency Medicine." *eMedicine–Medical Reference*. WebMD, 1 Apr. 2010. Web, 15 June 2010. http://emedicine.medscape .com/article/777026-overview.

97   "Pubococcygeus Muscle." *Livestrong.com*. Web, 15 June 2010. http:// www.livestrong.com/pubococcygeus-muscle/.

98   "Kegel Exercises." *Kegel Exercises for Men*. Web, 15 June 2010. http:// www.kegelexercisesformen.com/kegel_exercises_for_men.html.

99   "Erectile Dysfunction: A Sign of Heart Disease?" *MayoClinic.com*. 14 May 2010. Web, 15 June 2010. http://www.mayoclinic.com/health/ erectile-dysfunction/HB00074.

100   "Zinc Information Sheet." *The Vegetarian Society*. Web, 15 June 2010. http://www.vegsoc.org/info/zinc.html.

101   Leech, Eric. "8 Vitamins and Herbs To Improve Your Sex Life Naturally." *Planet Green*. 16 Dec. 2008. Web, 15 June 2010. http://planetgreen.discovery.com/food-health/vitamins-herbs -sex-life.html.

102   Roland, James. "Vitamins for Male Erection." *LiveStrong.com*. 19 Apr. 2010. Web, 15 June 2010. http://www.livestrong.com/ article/108807-vitamins-male-erection/.

103   "5 Medication-Free Strategies to Help Prevent Heart Disease." *MayoClinic.com*. 15 Jan. 1999. Web, 15 June 2010. http://www .mayoclinic.com/health/heart-disease-prevention/WO00041.

104   Kellogg, John Harvey. *Plain Facts for Old and Young*. Burlington, Iowa: I.F. Segner, 1882. Print, p. 356.

105   Leitzmann, MF, EA Pltaz, MJ Stampfer, WC Willett, and E. Giovannucci. "Ejaculation Frequency and Subsequent Risk of Prostate Cancer." *The Journal of the American Medical Association* 291.13 (2004): 1578-586. *PubMed.gov*. Web, 15 June 2010. http://www.ncbi.nlm.nih .gov/pubmed/15069045.

106   Giles, GG, G. Severi, DR English, MR McCredie, R. Borland, P. Boyle, and JL Hopper. "Sexual Factors and Prostate Cancer." *BJU International* 92.3 (2003): 211-16. *PubMed.gov*. Web, 15 June 2010. http://www.ncbi.nlm.nih.gov/pubmed/12887469.

107   Adelaide, Douglas Fox. "Masturbating May Protect against Prostate Cancer–16 July 2003–New Scientist." *New Scientist*. 16 July 2003. Web, 15 June 2010. http://www.newscientist.com/article/dn3942 -masturbating-may-protect-against-prostate-cancer.html.

108   "Urban Dictionary: DSB." *Urban Dictionary*. 30 June 2004. Web, 15 June 2010. http://www.urbandictionary.com/define.php?term =DSB&defid=741262.

109   "ACS Overview: Prostate Cancer." *American Cancer Society*. Web, 15 June 2010. http://www.cancer.org/docroot/CRI/CRI_2_1x .asp?rnav=criov&dt=36.

ACKNOWLEDGEMENTS

First, we'd like to thank all of the collective penises we've played with over the years. You all have given us quite a few thrills, chills, tasty snacks, and fun rides. We have yet to meet a penis we don't like (although some of the men attached to those cocks are sometimes not as charming as their parts). We'd also like to thank all of the men and women who participated in our surveys—by sharing your utmost private details with us, you contributed greatly to the content of this book. Thank you to our dear male friends who have put up with more than your share of pestering, intimate questions, and special thanks goes to our partners and lovers, Joe and Tre'. Thank you to Jill Alexander for being an amazingly patient, helpful, and understanding editor, as well as to John Gettings. You both kept us on track and helped shape this book into the fun, sexy guide it is. Thank you, Emmanuelle, for being our shining star and never-failing advocate. And finally, thank you to our parents, who taught us that it's okay to laugh about sex.